Workbook for

The Nursing Assistant's Handbook

By Hartman Publishing, Inc.

SECOND EDITION

Credits

MANAGING EDITOR
Susan Alvare

COVER DESIGNER
Kirsten Browne

INTERIOR DESIGNER/ILLUSTRATOR
Thaddeus Castillo

COMPOSITION
Thaddeus Castillo

PROOFREADERS
Suzanne Wegner
Jennifer Meehan
Michele Wiedemer

Notice to Readers

Though the guidelines and procedures contained in this text are based on consultations with healthcare professionals, they should not be considered absolute recommendations. The instructor and readers should follow employer, local, state, and federal guidelines concerning healthcare practices. These guidelines change, and it is the reader's responsibility to be aware of these changes and of the policies and procedures of her or his healthcare facility. The publisher, author, editors, and reviewers cannot accept any responsibility for errors or omissions or for any consequences from application of the information in this book and make no warranty, expressed or implied, with respect to the contents of the book. The Publisher does not warrant or guarantee any of the products described herein or perform any analysis in connection with any of the product information contained herein.

Copyright Information

preface

Welcome to the Workbook!

This workbook is designed to help you review what you have learned from reading your textbook. For this reason, the workbook is organized around learning objectives, just like your textbook and even your instructor's teaching material. Including the learning objectives makes it easier for you to go back and reread a section if you need to refresh your memory.

These learning objectives work as a built-in study guide. After completing the exercises for each learning objective in the workbook, ask yourself if you can DO what that learning objective describes.

If you can, move on to the next learning objective. If you cannot, just go back to the textbook, reread that learning objective, and try again.

We have provided procedure checklists near the end of the workbook. The answers to the workbook exercises are in your instructor's teaching guide.

Happy Learning!

table of contents

one

Long-Term Care and the Nursing Assistant's Role

Unit 1. Compare long-term care to other healthcare settings

Matching.

Write the letter of the correct definition beside each term listed at right.

a. Care provided in a person's home

b. Care performed in hospitals for temporary, but serious, illnesses or injuries

c. Care performed by a specially-trained therapist to restore or improve function after an illness or injury

d. Short-term care usually provided for less than 24 hours for persons who have had treatments or surgery

e. Care provided for persons who need some help with daily care and possibly medications, but do not need skilled care

f. Care for persons who have six months or less to live

g. Persons who live in nursing homes

h. Care in a hospital or nursing home for persons who need more observation and care than some long-term care facilities can offer

i. 24-hour care and help for long-term conditions; other terms for this type of care are nursing homes or extended care facilities

j. Care given at a facility during daytime work hours; generally, it is for people who need some help but are not seriously ill or disabled

k. Conditions that last a long period of time.

1. _____ Acute care

2. _____ Assisted living

3. _____ Home health care

4. _____ Hospice

5. _____ Outpatient care

6. _____ Rehabilitation

7. _____ Chronic

8. _____ Subacute care

9. _____ Long-term care

10. _____ Residents

11. _____ Adult daycare

Unit 2. Describe a typical long-term care facility

True or False.

Mark each statement with either a "T" for true or an "F" for false.

1. _____ LTC facilities do not have dementia units.

2. _____ When specialized care is offered in a LTC facility, employees may have special training.

3. _____ Subacute care is never offered in a LTC facility.

4. _____ Nonprofit organizations can own LTC facilities.

Unit 3. Explain Medicare and Medicaid

Fill in the Blank.

Write the correct answer in the blanks below.

1. CMS runs two national healthcare programs:_____
_____.

2. Medicare is a health insurance program for people _____ years old or older. It also covers people who are
_____
_____.

3. Medicare and Medicaid both help pay for _____ and
_____
for millions of Americans.

4. The Centers for Medicare & Medicaid Services (CMS) was formerly called the
_____
_____.

5. Medicaid is a medical assistance program for _____ people.

6. Medicare and Medicaid pay long-term care facilities a _____ amount for services for residents.

Unit 4. Describe the role of the nursing assistant

Short Answer.

1. Why is a nursing assistant one of the most important members of the care team?
_____
_____
_____
_____

2. List three tasks nursing assistants are usually NOT allowed to do.
_____
_____
_____
_____
_____
_____

3. What is charting?
_____
_____
_____
_____

Unit 5. Describe the care team and the chain of command

Crossword.

Clues:

Across

2. Abbreviation for one type of nurse who passes medications and performs treatments
_____

6. A _____ language pathologist evaluates a person's ability to swallow food and drink.
_____

7. An occupational therapist helps residents learn to compensate for these:
_____

8. Developed for each resident to achieve certain goals
_____

9. Person who diagnoses disease or disability and prescribes treatment
_____

Down

1. Defines the things NAs are allowed to do and how to do them correctly

   _____

3. One role of this person is to write and develop a care plan for each resident.

   _____

4. Helps residents with social needs, such as locating clothing if the resident's family is not involved

   _____

5. Term describing the line of authority in a facility

   _____

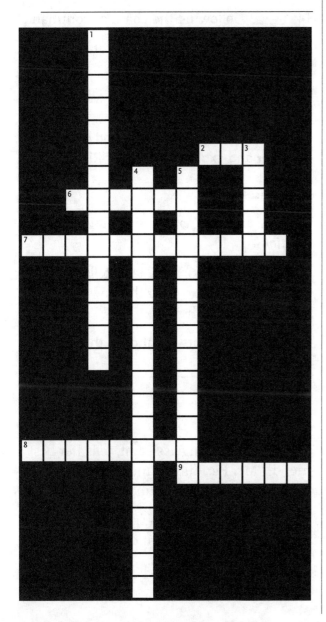

Labeling.

Fill in the blanks of the chain of command with members of the care team. Some have already been filled in for you.

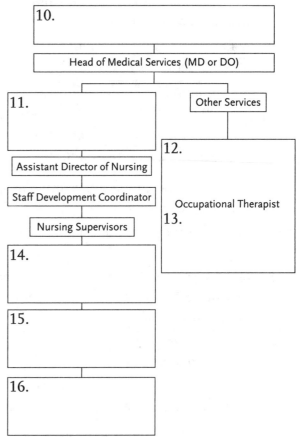

Unit 6. Define policies, procedures and professionalism

Multiple Choice.

Circle the letter of the answer that best completes the statement or answers the question.

1. Examples of common policies at facilities include all of the following EXCEPT:

   a. Keeping all resident information confidential

   b. Following the resident's care plan

   c. Discussing troubles at home with residents

   d. Performing only tasks that are included in your job description

2. Which of the following is NOT an example of having a professional relationship with a resident?

   a. Asking a resident, "Can you give me a few minutes? I've just had a fight with my boyfriend."

   b. Asking, "Mr. Gomez, would you mind if I entered your room?"

   c. Listening to Ms. Petrie while she talks about a loved one's death.

   d. Explaining to Mrs. Olsen about the bath you are going to give her.

3. Which of the following is an example of compassionate behavior?

   a. Making fun of Mrs. Klepstein's baggy sweater.

   b. Making sure that other people cannot see your resident while you are helping her dress.

   c. Telling other staff about a resident who cried in front of you.

   d. Laughing when a resident tells you she thinks she is very sick.

4. Being respectful towards a resident includes:

   a. Telling her that you do not like the cross she wears around her neck

   b. Asking her to believe in God if she does not

   c. Telling her who to vote for in the upcoming election

   d. Calling her by the name she wishes to be called

Short Answer.

Mark an "X" by all examples of a professional relationship with an employer.

5. _____ Completing duties efficiently

6. _____ Deciding for yourself when you should and should not follow policies and procedures

7. _____ Always documenting and reporting carefully and correctly

8. _____ Keeping problems you have with residents a secret

9. _____ Never asking questions when you do not know or understand something

10. _____ Taking directions or criticism without getting upset

11. _____ Being clean and neatly dressed

12. _____ Being late for work

13. _____ Forgetting to call in if you cannot make it to work

14. _____ Following the chain of command

15. _____ Participating in education programs

16. _____ Being a positive role model

Unit 7. List examples of legal and ethical behavior and explain Residents' Rights

Case Studies.

Read the following sentences and answer the questions.

Matt, a new nursing assistant, tells a resident that she has to wear the flowered shirt he picked out for her.

1. Which residents' right does this violate?

_____

_____

Margaret, a nursing assistant, tells her best friend, "Ms. Picadilly's cancer is getting worse. I heard her moaning all night last night."

2. Which residents' right does this violate?

_____

_____

_____

_____

Harry, a nursing assistant, is taking vital signs on his resident when the resident's family arrives. He tells them, "You'll have to come back another day. I'm busy with her right now."

3. Which residents' right does this violate?

_____

_____

_____

Yvonne, a nursing assistant, is going off duty. Leaving Ms. Rice's room, she notices a pretty necklace. She decides to borrow it for the night, promising to herself to return it tomorrow. She knows Ms. Rice has Alzheimer's and won't notice that it is gone anyway.

4. Which residents' right does this violate?

_____

_____

_____

Jane is explaining a care procedure to Mrs. Gonzalez in English. Mrs. Gonzalez only speaks Spanish. When she is finished, Jane asks Mrs. Gonzalez if she understands the procedure. Mrs. Gonzalez looks confused and doesn't respond. Jane begins to perform the care on Mrs. Gonzalez.

5. Which residents' right does this violate?

_____

_____

_____

_____

_____

_____

You are the nursing assistant for a resident who is paralyzed on her right side from a recent stroke. Some of her family members are visiting and one of them turns to you and says in a loud voice, "She looks so stupid with half of her face drooping down like that. Isn't there something you can do to fix that?"

6. What kind of abuse is this?
    a. Physical abuse
    b. Psychological abuse
    c. Invasion of privacy
    d. Financial abuse

You see a nursing assistant slap a resident with dementia on the hand because she is yelling and refusing to let the nursing assistant bathe her.

7. What kind of abuse is this?
    a. Physical abuse
    b. Psychological abuse
    c. Neglect
    d. Domestic violence

8. If a nursing assistant suspects an elderly resident is being abused, the NA must:
    a. Ask another resident if he thinks that person is being abused
    b. Ask his family and friends for advice
    c. Report it to his supervisor and let her handle it from there
    d. Do nothing since someone has probably already reported it

9. Which of the following responses is true of OBRA?
    a. Nursing assistants must have 150 hours of training.
    b. OBRA was passed in 1977.
    c. Nursing assistants must pass a competency evaluation before being employed.
    d. Residents' Rights are not a part of OBRA.

10. Which of the following is a requirement of HIPAA?

    a. Nursing assistants can give out resident information to anyone who asks for it.

    b. Health information must be kept private.

    c. There are no penalties for not following HIPAA guidelines.

    d. Doctors do not need to follow HIPAA rules.

11. Protected health information includes

    a. Food preferences

    b. Favorite activities

    c. Personal possessions

    d. Social security numbers

Matching.

Write the letter of the correct definition beside each term listed at the right.

a. Forcing a person to perform or participate in sexual acts.

b. Stealing, taking advantage of, or improperly using the money, property, or other assets of another person.

c. Actually touching a person without his permission.

d. The use of legal or illegal drugs, cigarettes or alcohol in a way that harms oneself or others.

e. Abuse by spouses, intimate partners, or family members.

f. Abuse of staff by residents or other staff members.

g. Confining or separating a person from others in a certain area.

h. Harming a person by failing to give needed care.

i. Emotionally harming a person by threatening, scaring, humiliating, intimidating, isolating, insulting, or treating him or her as a child.

j. Any treatment, intentional or not, that causes harm to a person's body.

k. Threatening and making a person feel fearful that he or she will be touched without permission.

l. Unlawful restraint of someone that affects the person's freedom of movement; includes threat of restraint and actual restraint.

m. Unwelcome sexual advances or behavior that creates an intimidating or offensive working environment.

n. Violating someone's right to privacy by exposing his or her private affairs, name, or photograph to the public without consent.

o. Purposely causing physical, mental, or emotional pain or injury to someone.

12. _____ Abuse

13. _____ Neglect

14. _____ Physical abuse

15. _____ Sexual abuse

16. _____ Psychological abuse

17. _____ Financial abuse

18. _____ Assault

19. _____ Battery

20. _____ Domestic violence

21. _____ Workplace violence

22. _____ False imprisonment

23. _____ Involuntary seclusion

24. _____ Sexual harassment

25. _____ Substance abuse

26. _____ Invasion of privacy

Unit 8. Explain legal aspects of the resident's medical record

Short Answer.

1. List the four reasons why careful documentation is important.

   _____

   _____

   _____

   _____

   _____

   _____

   _____

   _____

   _____

2. Why should nursing assistants write notes immediately after giving care?

   _____

   _____

   _____

   _____

   _____

3. Change the following hours from regular time into military time:

   3:00 p.m.

   _____

   7:00 p.m.

   _____

   11:30 p.m.

   _____

4. Change the following hours from military time to standard time:

   1900 hours

   _____

   1600 hours

   _____

Unit 9. Explain the Minimum Data Set (MDS)

Short Answer.

1. How does a nursing assistant's reporting affect the MDS?

   _____

   _____

   _____

   _____

2. Why should nursing assistants always report any changes in a resident to the nurse?

   _____

   _____

   _____

3. How soon after a resident is admitted does an MDS on that resident need to be completed?

   _____

   _____

two

Foundations of Resident Care

Unit 1. Understand the importance of verbal and written communications

Multiple Choice.

Circle the letter of the answer that best completes the statement or answers the question.

1. Which of the following is an example of verbal communication?

    a. Telling a joke

    b. Smiling at a joke

2. Which of the following is an example of nonverbal communication?

    a. Asking for a glass of water

    b. Pointing to a glass of water

3. Types of verbal communication include:

    a. Writing

    b. Nodding your head

    c. Pointing

    d. Shrugging your shoulders

4. Types of nonverbal communication include:

    a. Speaking

    b. Facial expressions

    c. The way you say something

    d. Oral reports

5. Which of the following is an example of a confusing or conflicting message (saying one thing and meaning another)?

    a. Mr. Carter smiles happily and tells you he is excited because his daughter is coming to visit.

    b. Mrs. Sanchez looks like she is in pain. When you ask her about it, she tells you that her back has been bothering her lately.

    c. Ms. Jones agrees with you when you say it is a nice day, but she looks angry.

    d. Mr. Wilson won't watch his favorite TV show. He says he feels a little depressed.

Labeling.

Looking at the diagram, list examples of observations using each sense.

6. Smell:

    _____
    _____
    _____
    _____
    _____

7. Sight:

    _____
    _____
    _____
    _____
    _____

8. Hearing:

    _____
    _____
    _____
    _____
    _____

9. Touch:

    _____
    _____
    _____
    _____
    _____

Name: _____

Subjective or Objective?

For each of the following, decide whether it is an objective observation (you can see, hear, smell, or touch it) or subjective observation (the resident must tell you about it). Write "O" for objective and "S" for subjective.

10. _____ Skin rash

11. _____ Crying

12. _____ Rapid pulse

13. _____ Headache

14. _____ Nausea

15. _____ Vomiting

16. _____ Swelling

17. _____ Cloudy urine

18. _____ Depression

19. _____ Redness

20. _____ Fever

21. _____ Dizziness

22. _____ Noisy breathing

23. _____ Chest pain

24. _____ Toothache

25. _____ Coughing

26. _____ Painful breathing

27. _____ Fruity breath

28. _____ Itching

Short Answer.

29. What is a root?

_____

_____

30. What is a prefix?

_____

_____

31. What is a suffix?

_____

_____

Unit 2. Describe barriers to communication

Word Search.

s	t	o	v	a	f	p	o	f	w	z	a	s	z
l	y	v	o	s	b	s	w	c	z	d	l	o	m
a	c	o	y	z	i	z	i	l	v	o	g	m	h
n	i	l	o	x	g	g	a	i	w	d	w	k	t
g	r	o	i	n	d	n	c	l	s	a	p	h	s
s	u	c	y	c	g	e	y	e	u	h	l	q	d
e	o	p	k	u	h	o	f	l	n	l	j	f	o
k	p	j	a	h	e	e	p	e	x	e	w	v	y
q	w	g	f	r	u	z	s	i	l	h	g	z	f
h	e	q	k	x	q	x	i	t	n	p	s	o	y
k	r	n	t	x	f	q	g	g	d	i	m	e	l
r	x	n	x	u	o	l	x	e	h	f	o	i	o
f	p	u	h	u	s	g	k	l	f	z	u	n	s
x	f	x	n	u	b	s	t	n	e	i	t	a	p

Complete each of the following sentences and find your answers in the word search.

1. Do not offer your personal

   _____

   to the resident or give

   _____.

2. _____ words or expressions may not be understood and are unprofessional.

3. _____ are phrases that don't really mean anything.

4. Be _____ with a resident who is difficult to understand.

5. If a resident does not hear you or does not understand you, speak more

   _____.

6. If a resident does not understand you, speak in _____, everyday words.

Name: _____

7. Each person's background, values, and

_____

affect communication.

Unit 3. List guidelines for communicating with residents with special needs

Nursing assistant Mark Hedman is about to provide care for hearing-impaired resident Mrs. Castillo. She is standing at the window looking out at the gardens. He enters her room and asks if she would like her hair shampooed. She doesn't answer. He taps her on the back, and she jumps. He yells, "I said, 'Would you like to have your hair shampooed now?'"

1. What would have been a correct way for Mark to communicate with Mrs. Castillo?

_____
_____
_____
_____
_____
_____
_____
_____

Vision-impaired resident Ms. Crawford is being helped into a fellow resident's room for a visit. Nursing assistant Virginia Davies assists her to the door and says, "See you later, Ms. Crawford. I'll be back in about an hour to help you return to your room." Ms. Crawford enters the room, walks into a chair and almost falls over.

2. What would have been a correct way for Virginia to communicate with Ms. Crawford?

_____
_____

_____
_____
_____
_____

Kelley, a nursing assistant, is taking care of a mentally ill resident who is very withdrawn. Kelley moves around the room picking up clutter and saying to her resident in a bored tone: "How are we doing today, Mrs. Rogers? Are we going to start talking to Kelley today, or are we going to be quiet like we were yesterday?"

3. What would have been a correct way for Kelley to communicate with Mrs. Rogers?

_____
_____
_____
_____
_____
_____

Resident Joe Morteno has dementia and can be combative at times. On this particular day he lashes out at nursing assistant Serena Jones. "Why are you so stupid? You never understand what I really need," he yells. Serena replies, "I'm not stupid. You're the one who is stupid."

4. What would have been a correct way for Serena to communicate with Mr. Morteno?

_____
_____
_____
_____
_____
_____

Name: _____

Resident Kim Singer has dementia. One morning she starts touching herself when Joan, a nursing assistant, walks by. Joan yells, "Stop that right now! That is inappropriate!"

5. What would have been the correct way for Joan to respond to this behavior?

_____

_____

_____

_____

_____

_____

Unit 4. Identify ways to promote safety and handle non-medical emergencies

Short Answer.

1. Looking at the illustrations below, which drawing shows the correct way to lift objects? Why is it correct?

_____

_____

_____

_____

_____

_____

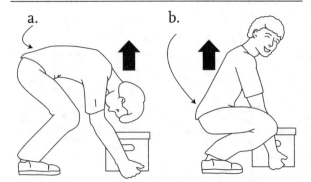

2. Why should an NA arrange a signal, such as counting to three, when moving a resident?

_____

_____

_____

True or False.

Mark each statement with either a "T" for true or an "F" for false.

3. _____ Applying the principles of good body mechanics to work can help avoid injury and save energy.

4. _____ To guard against choking, residents should eat sitting as upright as possible.

5. _____ To lift a heavy object from the floor, first place your feet together and keep your knees straight.

6. _____ The muscles of the thighs, upper arms, and shoulders should not be used to lift objects from the floor.

7. _____ Thickened liquids are harder to swallow.

8. _____ To help guard against falls, clear all walkways of clutter, throw rugs, and cords.

9. _____ Standing with legs shoulder-width apart gives a greater base of support.

10. _____ When moving an object, pivot your feet instead of twisting at the waist.

11. _____ It is a good idea to hold objects away from the body when lifting or carrying them.

12. _____ Never try to catch a falling resident as you could seriously injure yourself and/or the resident.

13. _____ Bending from the waist, rather than bending your knees, allows use of big muscles in the legs and hips rather than the smaller muscles in the back.

14. _____ Always check water temperature with a water thermometer or on your wrist before using it.

15. _____ Keeping call lights within a resident's reach can help guard against falls.

16. _____ If your clothing catches fire, run quickly to the nearest exit.

17. _____ Hot drinks should be placed on the edges of tables.

18. _____ Residents must be identified before helping with feeding or placing meal trays.

19. _____ The MSDS details chemical ingredients and chemical dangers of products.

20. _____ Residents do not need to be identified before performing care.

Short Answer.

Fill in the meanings of the following two acronyms.

21. To operate a fire extinguisher:

P _____

_____

A _____

_____

S _____

_____

S _____

_____

22. In case of a fire:

R _____

_____

A _____

_____

C _____

_____

E _____

_____

Labeling.

Looking at the illustration below, fill in the three parts of the ABC's of good body mechanics.

23.

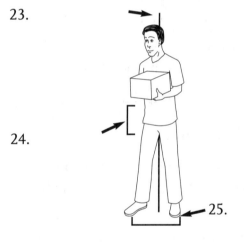

24.

25.

Unit 5. Demonstrate how to recognize and respond to medical emergencies

Short Answer.

1. When coming upon an emergency situation, what two important steps should be followed first?

_____

_____

_____

_____

Name: _____

Matching.

Write the letter of the correct definition beside each term listed below.

a. Signs of this include pale or bluish skin, staring, increased pulse and respiration rate, low blood pressure, and extreme thirst.

b. Signs of this include severe pain in the chest, anxiety, and indigestion.

c. Care given in an emergency before trained medical professionals can take over.

d. The name for the condition in which something is blocking the tube through which air enters the lungs.

e. An accident or an unexpected event during the course of care.

f. Apply firm pressure on the wound with a pad or clean cloth when this occurs.

g. If a person is sitting, have her bend forward and place her head between her knees before this occurs.

h. Signs that this is occurring include dizziness, ringing in the ears, blurred vision, and slurring of words.

i. Do not try to force anything, including your hands, in a person's mouth when this is happening.

j. Medical procedures used when a person's heart or lungs have stopped working.

k. Sweet or fruity breath is a symptom.

l. This can result from either too much insulin or too little food.

2. _____ Heart attack

3. _____ Bleeding

4. _____ CPR

5. _____ Shock

6. _____ Fainting

7. _____ Obstructed airway

8. _____ Stroke

9. _____ Seizure

10. _____ Diabetic coma

11. _____ Insulin shock

12. _____ First aid

13. _____ Incident

Unit 6. Describe and demonstrate infection control practices

Multiple Choice.

Circle the letter of the answer that best completes the statement or answers the question.

1. Which of the following statements is true of microorganisms?

    a. They are the set of methods to control the spread of disease.

    b. They are tiny living things always present in the environment.

    c. They are always harmful.

    d. They refer to a condition that means no pathogens are present.

2. An infection specifically acquired in a hospital or other healthcare facility is called a:

    a. Nosocomial infection

    b. Chain of infection

    c. Microorganism

    d. Localized infection

3. The following are necessary links in the chain of infection. By wearing gloves, which link is broken and thus prevents the spread of disease?

    a. Reservoir (place where the pathogen lives and grows)

    b. Mode of transmission (a way for the disease to spread)

Name: _____

c. Susceptible host (person who is likely to get the disease)

d. Portal of exit (body opening that allows pathogens to leave)

4. The following are necessary links in the chain of infection. By getting a vaccination shot for Hepatitis B, which link will be affected to prevent you from getting Hepatitis B?

a. Reservoir (place where the pathogen lives and grows)

b. Mode of transmission (a way for the disease to spread)

c. Susceptible host (person who is likely to get the disease)

d. Portal of exit (body opening that allows pathogens to leave)

5. Standard Precautions should be practiced:

a. Only on people who look like they have a bloodborne disease

b. On every single person in your care

c. Only on people who request that you follow them

d. On nobody in your care

6. Under Standard Precautions, "body fluids" do NOT include:

a. Sweat

b. Urine

c. Pus

d. Vaginal secretions

7. Standard Precautions include the following measures:

a. Not wearing gloves while shaving residents

b. Capping needles

c. Touching body fluids with bare hands

d. Washing hands before putting on and after removing gloves

8. The most important thing an NA can do to prevent the spread of disease is to:

a. Carry dirty linen close to the uniform

b. Never change gloves

c. Remove gloves before cleaning spills

d. Wash hands

9. Which of the following statements is true of hand hygiene?

a. Hand hygiene means never having to use soap and water for handwashing.

b. Hand hygiene eliminates all bacteria on the hands.

c. Hand hygiene means using soap and water, along with alcohol-based rubs.

d. Hand hygiene means do not use soap and water for visibly soiled hands.

Short Answer.

Mark an "X" next to the tasks that require the use of gloves.

10. _____ Handling body fluids

11. _____ Moving a resident's picture

12. _____ Anytime you may touch blood

13. _____ Combing a resident's hair

14. _____ Assisting with perineal care

15. _____ Giving a massage to a resident with broken skin on his back

16. _____ Performing mouth care

17. _____ Shaving a resident

18. What should a nursing assistant always do before and after wearing gloves?

_____

_____

_____

_____

Name: _____

19. After giving care to a resident, why should an NA remove her gloves before leaving the room?

_____

_____

_____

_____

20. Why do you think PPE is so important in the healthcare setting?

_____

_____

_____

21. When putting on PPE, what is the correct order?

1st _____

2nd _____

3rd _____

22. When removing PPE, what is the correct order?

1st _____

2nd _____

3rd _____

True or False.

Mark each statement with either a "T" for true or an "F" for false.

23. _____ Sterilization means only pathogens are destroyed.

24. _____ Roll linens so that the dirtiest area is inside.

25. _____ If broken glass is present, you can pick up large pieces with your hands.

26. _____ When handling soiled linens, keep them close to your uniform.

27. _____ Practicing Transmission-Based Precautions means NAs do not have to follow Standard Precautions.

28. _____ Airborne Precautions are used when a microorganism does not stay suspended in the air.

29. _____ Laughing and sneezing can generate droplets.

30. _____ Tuberculosis is an example of an airborne disease.

31. _____ Contact Precautions include not touching an infected surface without wearing gloves.

32. _____ Hepatitis B is a bloodborne disease.

33. _____ Employers offer a free vaccine for hepatitis B.

34. _____ Tuberculosis cannot be cured.

35. _____ MRSA is most often spread by direct physical contact.

36. _____ VRE can be controlled by antibiotics.

37. _____ Proper handwashing is one of the most important ways to prevent the spread of VRE and MRSA.

38. _____ The overuse of antibiotics can increase the risk of developing C. difficile.

39. _____ Employers are not required to provide PPE for employees to use.

Name: _____

three

Understanding Your Residents

Unit 1. Explain why promoting independence and self-care is important

Word Search.

Complete each of the following sentences and find your answers in the word search.

d	a	s	b	e	k	z	l	v	f	o	i	e	d
b	e	d	k	l	c	g	g	b	j	n	l	r	z
c	v	s	r	x	x	n	v	q	d	h	b	a	u
y	a	b	b	d	d	z	e	e	w	c	k	c	f
t	m	s	e	v	u	k	p	d	i	z	v	f	h
h	x	z	b	n	p	e	u	f	n	n	i	l	t
g	q	o	p	h	n	i	k	k	v	e	v	e	w
p	y	t	o	d	n	o	e	s	t	y	p	s	z
l	l	s	e	i	t	i	v	i	t	c	a	e	t
h	z	n	z	v	c	p	x	t	p	o	y	h	d
f	c	c	m	j	d	d	f	y	f	u	a	n	u
e	l	b	p	d	x	g	o	x	w	v	t	w	p
g	w	w	y	i	i	h	l	u	j	j	w	p	w
c	w	d	y	e	z	d	h	g	s	g	d	m	e

1. A loss of _____ is very difficult for a person to deal with.

2. Allow a resident to do a _____ independently even if it's easier for you to do it.

3. _____ of daily living (ADLs) are personal care tasks done every day to care for yourself.

4. Encourage _____, regardless of how long it takes or how poorly they do it.

5. A loss of independence can cause increased _____ _____.

Case Study.

Read the following paragraph and answer the question below.

Sarah, a nursing assistant, is assisting resident Mrs. Sanchez today. It is time to get Mrs. Sanchez dressed and ready for breakfast. Sarah enters the room without knocking. She doesn't see Mrs. Sanchez. She walks over to the bathroom door and opens it. Mrs. Sanchez is pulling up her underpants. "Hurry up," says Sarah. "We've got to get you dressed."

Sarah chooses and lays out clean clothes. Mrs. Sanchez starts to take off her nightgown but has trouble getting it over her head. Sarah impatiently reaches over and yanks it over her head. "Sit down. It will be faster if I do this." She quickly starts putting a clean shirt on Mrs. Sanchez.

6. List all of the examples of how Sarah did NOT promote privacy, dignity, and independence.

_____

_____

_____

_____

_____

_____

_____

Name: _____

Short Answer.

7. Write a brief paragraph explaining everything you did this morning before arriving in class. Include things such as bathing, going to the bathroom, applying makeup, brushing your hair, brushing your teeth, walking around your house, etc. Then answer question #8 below.

_____

_____

_____

_____

_____

_____

_____

_____

8. How would you feel if you were unable to do one or more of the tasks above by yourself?

_____

_____

_____

_____

_____

_____

_____

Unit 2. Identify basic human needs

Multiple Choice.

Circle the letter of the answer that best completes the statement or answers the question.

1. Basic physical needs include:
   a. Need for self-esteem
   b. Food and water
   c. Social interaction with others
   d. Psychosocial needs

2. If an NA encounters a resident in a sexual situation, she should:
   a. Provide privacy
   b. Tell the resident that what he is doing is wrong
   c. Tell another nursing assistant that the resident is disgusting
   d. Ask him to stop

3. Psychosocial needs include the following:
   a. Love and affection
   b. Sleep and rest
   c. Food
   d. Water

Short Answer.

Mark an "X" next to examples of good ways to assist residents with their spiritual needs.

4. _____ A resident tells you that he cannot drink milk with his hamburger due to his religious beliefs. He asks you for some water instead. You notify the nurse, take the milk away, and bring him some water.

5. _____ A resident tells you she is a Baptist and wants to know when the next Baptist service will be. "A Baptist?" you ask. "Why don't you just attend a Catholic service? One is starting in ten minutes."

6. _____ A resident asks you to read a passage from his Bible. He tells you that it will comfort him. You open the Bible and begin to read.

7. _____ A resident wants to see a rabbi. You report this request to the nurse.

8. _____ You see a Buddha statue in a resident's room. You laugh and tell the resident, "I couldn't keep this thing next to my bed. It would make me laugh too much."

9. _____ A spiritual leader is visiting with a resident. You quietly leave the room and shut the door.

10. _____ A resident tells you he is Muslim. You begin to explain Christianity to him and ask him to attend a Presbyterian service just to see what it's like.

11. _____ A resident tells you that she does not believe in God. You do believe in God but do not argue with her. You listen quietly as she tells you her reasons.

Labeling.

Fill in the following blanks to complete the types of needs in "Maslow's Hierarchy of Needs."

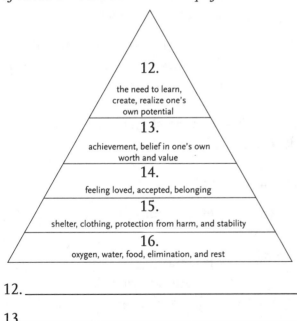

12. the need to learn, create, realize one's own potential

13. achievement, belief in one's own worth and value

14. feeling loved, accepted, belonging

15. shelter, clothing, protection from harm, and stability

16. oxygen, water, food, elimination, and rest

12._____

13._____

14._____

15._____

16._____

Unit 3. Identify ways to accommodate cultural differences

Crossword.

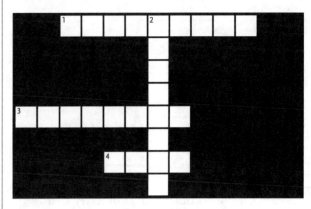

Clues:

Across

1. Cultural _____ has to do with a variety of people who live and work together in the world.

   _____

3. An interpreter can help you understand this if a resident speaks a different one than you do.

   _____

4. Religious beliefs may include restrictions on this and must be respected.

   _____

Down

2. When people are ill or dying, this may become especially important.

   _____

Short Answer.

5. Briefly describe the culture in which you grew up.

   _____

   _____

   _____

_____
_____
_____
_____
_____
_____

Unit 4. Describe the need for activity

Short Answer.

List seven ways that regular activity can help a person.

_____
_____
_____
_____
_____
_____
_____

Unit 5. Discuss family roles and their significance in health care

Short Answer.

1. List four ways families help residents in long-term care.

_____
_____
_____
_____
_____

2. What is some important information that family members can contribute about residents?

_____
_____
_____
_____

True or False.

Mark each statement with either a "T" for true or an "F" for false.

3. _____ It is okay to discuss any medical information about a resident with his family members.

4. _____ A family can be an unmarried couple.

5. _____ Families play a huge role in most people's lives.

6. _____ Do not ask a family member questions about when a resident likes to eat breakfast.

7. _____ It is not necessary to report abusive behavior from a family member to the nurse.

Unit 6. Describe the stages of human development

Fill in the Blank.

1. Infants develop from the _____ down.

2. Toddlers learn to _____, gain coordination of their limbs, and control their bladders and bowels.

3. Children in their preschool years begin to learn right from _____.

4. School-age children develop a conscience, morals, and

_____.

5. _____ occurs between the ages of 10 to 16 for girls and ages 12 to 14 for boys.

6. Adolescents are concerned with

    _____

    image and acceptance by their peers.

7. Young adults may select a _____.

8. Ideas about older adults are often

    _____.

9. Prejudice toward the elderly is called

    _____.

Short Answer.

10. In the movies and on television, older people are usually portrayed as slow, lonely, helpless, or dependent. However, this is often false. Can you think of a positive portrayal of an older person on television or in a movie? If so, list it here. Briefly describe what you like about the character.

    _____

    _____

    _____

    _____

    _____

Mark an "X" next to normal changes of aging.

11. _____ Depression

12. _____ Drier skin

13. _____ Mild forgetfulness

14. _____ Incontinence

15. _____ Poor nutrition

16. _____ Less efficient heart

17. _____ More frequent elimination

18. _____ Weaker muscles

Unit 7. Discuss the needs of people with developmental disabilities

Short Answer.

1. List three abilities that may be affected by developmental disabilities.

    _____

    _____

    _____

    _____

2. List four guidelines for caring for a resident who is developmentally disabled.

    _____

    _____

    _____

    _____

    _____

    _____

    _____

Unit 8. Explain how to care for dying residents

Multiple Choice.

Circle the letter of the answer that best completes the statement or answers the question.

1. Mrs. Levine, a resident, prays about her terminal illness. She promises God that she will make peace with her sister, whom she has not seen in 20 years, if she is allowed to live. Which stage of dying is Mrs. Levine going through?

    a. Denial

    b. Anger

    c. Bargaining

    d. Depression

    e. Acceptance

Name: _____

2. A terminally ill resident, Mr. Lucero, begins to yell at Peter, his nursing assistant. He says that he never took good care of him. He blames Peter for a lack of proper care. Peter does not take it personally because he realizes that Mr. Lucero may be going through the _____ stage of dying.

   a. Denial
   b. Anger
   c. Bargaining
   d. Depression
   e. Acceptance

3. Resident Wilda Scott is dying. Her priest visits her at her request. When he asks her if there is anything he can do to help her get things in order, she tells him she has no idea what he is talking about. Instead she begins to tell him the latest news about her son. Mrs. Scott is experiencing:

   a. Denial
   b. Anger
   c. Bargaining
   d. Depression
   e. Acceptance

4. A terminally ill resident, John Castillo, visits with his family. He discusses his funeral arrangements with them. He lets them know that he is concerned about their well-being after he is gone. He says he wants to spend as much time as possible with them before he dies. Mr. Castillo is going through the _____ stage of dying.

   a. Denial
   b. Anger
   c. Bargaining
   d. Depression
   e. Acceptance

5. A terminally ill resident cries constantly. She doesn't want to talk to anyone. She may be experiencing the _____ stage of dying.

   a. Denial
   b. Anger
   c. Bargaining
   d. Depression
   e. Acceptance

True or False.

Mark each statement with either a "T" for true or an "F" for false.

6. _____ Advance directives do not need to be honored if the medical professional feels he can save the resident's life.

7. _____ Listening to a resident who is dying is very important.

8. _____ All people grieve in the same way.

9. _____ Hearing is usually the last sense to leave the body.

10. _____ A person may be incontinent after death.

11. _____ Skin care is not important for a dying resident.

12. _____ Keep the room softly lighted for a dying resident.

13. _____ Blurred vision is a sign of approaching death.

14. _____ It is important to observe dying residents for signs of pain.

15. _____ Mouth care should not be given to dying residents.

16. _____ Residents do not have the right to refuse treatment when they are dying.

17. _____ Feelings about death can be influenced by a person's cultural background.

18. _____ It is best to isolate and avoid a dying resident.

19. _____ Do not make promises to dying residents that cannot or should not be kept.

20. _____ After a resident has died, do not remove tubes or any other equipment.

Unit 9. Define the goals of a hospice program

Short Answer.

1. How do the goals of hospice care differ from those of long-term care?

_____
_____
_____
_____
_____
_____
_____
_____
_____
_____

Fill in the Blank.

2. Hospice care uses a _____ approach.

3. Residents who are dying also need to feel _____ for as long as possible.

4. In hospice care, focus on relieving residents' _____ and making them comfortable rather than teaching them to care for themselves.

5. Recognize that some persons wish to be _____ with their dying loved ones.

6. Be a good _____ to a dying resident, and do not feel obligated to respond.

7. In hospice care, the type of care that focuses on the comfort and dignity of the resident is called _____ care.

four

Body Systems

Fill in the Blank.

1. The largest organ and system in the body is the _____.

2. Skin prevents the loss of too much _____, which is essential to life.

3. The skin is also a _____ organ that feels heat, cold, pain, touch, and pressure.

4. Muscles, bones, ligaments, tendons, and cartilage work together to allow the body to _____.

5. _____ is important for improving and maintaining physical and mental health.

6. When _____ develop, the muscle shortens, becomes inflexible, and "freezes" in position.

7. The nervous system is the _____ center and _____ center of the body.

8. The nervous system _____ and interprets information from the environment outside the body.

9. Eyes, ears, tongue, nose, and skin relay impulses to _____.

10. The circulatory system is made up of the _____, blood vessels, and _____.

11. Blood carries food, _____, and other needed substances to cells.

12. The circulatory system helps remove _____ products from cells.

13. The _____ accomplish the process of respiration.

14. Two functions of the respiratory system involve bringing oxygen into the body and eliminating _____.

15. The urinary system eliminates waste products created by the cells through _____.

16. The gastrointestinal system has two functions: _____ and _____.

17. The endocrine system is made up of glands that secrete _____.

18. Hormones regulate levels of _____ in the blood and _____ in the bones.

19. The function of the reproductive system is to allow human beings to _____, or create new human life.

20. Sex glands are called the _____.

21. The immune system protects the body from _____-causing bacteria, viruses, and organisms.

22. The lymphatic system removes excess _____ and waste products from the body's tissues.

True or False.

Looking at the normal changes of aging for each body system, mark each statement with either a "T" for true or an "F" for false.

23. _____ A normal change of aging for the integumentary system is that skin becomes thicker and more oily.

24. _____ An older person may feel colder because protective fatty tissue becomes thinner.

25. _____ A person may lose height as she ages.

26. _____ Bones become thicker and harder to break as a person ages.

27. _____ A normal change of aging for the nervous system is slower responses and reflexes.

28. _____ All older people will be extremely forgetful and unable to remember much of anything.

29. _____ As a person ages, he may find it harder to taste or smell foods.

30. _____ Narrowed blood vessels and decreased blood flow are normal changes of aging for the circulatory system.

31. _____ The strength of the lungs decreases as a person ages.

32. _____ The bladder holds more urine as a person ages, making urination less frequent.

33. _____ A normal change of aging for the urinary system is that the bladder may not empty completely. This makes the risk of infection higher.

34. _____ An older person may be constipated more often.

35. _____ As a person ages, she may have a decrease of saliva and other digestive fluids.

36. _____ The body becomes better able to handle stress with age.

37. _____ A decrease in progesterone and estrogen is a normal change of aging for the endocrine system.

38. _____ For women, aging means a higher risk of osteoporosis due to a loss of calcium from a decrease in estrogen.

39. _____ An older male will produce more sperm.

40. _____ An older person will be at a higher risk for all types of infections.

41. _____ A normal change of aging for the immune system is an increased response to vaccines.

Scenarios.

Read the following paragraphs and decide which items should be reported to the nurse.

Integumentary System

42. You are providing care for Mrs. Miller. As you are assisting her to turn over, you notice that she has a red spot above her buttocks and a bruise on her upper arm. Which items need to be reported to the nurse?

_____

_____

_____

Name: _____

_____
_____
_____
_____

Musculoskeletal System

43. You are providing care for Mr. Leary. As you assist him out of bed, he moves slowly. Today he could only walk a shorter distance than yesterday. He seems to be limping and occasionally makes a noise. Which items need to be reported to the nurse?

_____
_____
_____
_____
_____
_____

Nervous System

44. You are assisting Ms. Rice with eating. It takes her a few seconds to take the napkin you are offering her. While she is eating, you notice she coughs while swallowing. She suddenly says that she cannot see the food on the left side of her plate. Which items need to be reported to the nurse?

_____
_____
_____
_____
_____
_____

Circulatory System

45. You are giving Mrs. Lee a bed bath. You notice that her fingertips are blue and her feet are swollen. She complains of being tired. Which items need to be reported to the nurse?

_____
_____
_____
_____
_____
_____

Respiratory System

46. You are giving care to Mr. Martin. He makes a wheezing sound when he breathes out of his mouth. After turning over, he says he needs to rest before continuing. He begins to cough. Which items need to be reported to the nurse?

_____
_____
_____
_____
_____

Urinary System

47. You always need to give Mr. Parsons a urinal before and after you help him walk. Today you notice that his urine seems cloudy and foul-smelling. When you come in later, you find urine on his bed linens. Which items need to be reported to the nurse?

_____
_____
_____

Name: _____

_____
_____
_____
_____

Gastrointestinal System

48. Mr. Sanchez is not eating as much as he used to. He has lost two pounds since you last weighed him. He says he just isn't as hungry lately. Which items need to be reported to the nurse?

_____
_____
_____
_____
_____
_____
_____

Endocrine System

49. You walk into Mrs. Walker's room and notice she has just finished drinking her water from the glass beside her bed. She asks you to refill her water pitcher because it's empty. You just filled it ten minutes ago. When you return with her pitcher, you see that she is sweating even though she has no blanket over her and the room feels cool to you. Which items need to be reported to the nurse?

_____
_____
_____
_____
_____
_____

Reproductive System

50. You offer Mr. Tadley a urinal because he requests it. He has trouble urinating and his face indicates that he is in pain. He later tells you he has a sore area on his penis. Which items need to be reported to the nurse?

_____
_____
_____
_____
_____
_____
_____

Immune and Lymphatic Systems

51. Ms. Gallagher is running a fever. She complains of being tired and mentions that she has had three bouts of diarrhea in the last hour. Which items need to be reported to the nurse?

_____
_____
_____
_____

Short Answer.

For each body system, write down two ways NAs can help residents with their normal changes of aging. One example has been completed for you.

Integumentary System

1. Keep resident's skin clean and dry.

2. _____

_____

Name: _____

Musculoskeletal System

1. _____

_____

_____

_____

2. _____

_____

_____

_____

Nervous System

1. _____

_____

_____

_____

2. _____

_____

_____

_____

Circulatory System

1. _____

_____

_____

_____

2. _____

_____

_____

_____

Respiratory System

1. _____

_____

_____

2. _____

_____

_____

_____

Urinary System

1. _____

_____

_____

_____

2. _____

_____

_____

_____

Gastrointestinal System

1. _____

_____

_____

_____

2. _____

_____

_____

_____

Endocrine System

1. _____

_____

_____

_____

2. _____

_____

_____

_____

Reproductive System

1. _____

_____

_____

_____

2. _____

_____

_____

_____

Immune and Lymphatic Systems

1. _____

_____

_____

_____

2. _____

_____

_____

_____

Name: _____

five
Personal Care Skills

Unit 1. Explain personal care of residents

Fill in the Blank.

1. Tasks NAs assist with and how much help that is given will depend on a resident's

    _____

    to do self-care.

2. Personal care is a very

    _____

    experience.

3. Personal care may be

    _____

    for some residents.

4. Be _____
    when helping with personal care tasks.

5. Before you begin any task,

    _____

    to the resident exactly what you will be doing.

6. Ask if he or she would like to use the

    _____

    or bedpan first.

7. Provide the resident with

    _____.

8. During personal care,

    _____

    for any problems or changes that have occurred.

9. After care make sure the

    _____

    is within reach and the bed is left in its

    _____

    position.

10. If the resident seems tired, stop and take a short _____.

11. AM or PM care refers to the time of

    _____

    care tasks are performed.

Unit 2. Describe guidelines for assisting with bathing

True or False.

Mark each statement with either a "T" for true or an "F" for false.

1. _____ Older skin produces less perspiration and oil.

2. _____ Check to make sure the bathroom or shower room floor is dry before giving a shower or tub bath.

3. _____ The face, hands, underarms, and perineum should be washed once a week.

4. _____ Checking the water temperature before bathing is not necessary.

5. _____ Bathing provides a great opportunity to observe a resident's skin.

6. _____ Have the resident use safety bars when getting into or out of the tub or shower.

7. _____ Checking to make sure the room is warm enough for the resident before bathing is important.

8. _____ Use bath oils when assisting a resident to take a tub bath.

9. _____ Covering a resident while transporting to and from shower or tub room provides warmth and privacy.

10. _____ Leave the resident alone while he or she is in the shower room.

Short Answer.

11. Think about your own routine for bathing. If you were unable to do it by yourself, how would you feel? Why is protecting a resident's privacy so important when bathing?

_____

_____

_____

_____

_____

_____

_____

_____

_____

Unit 3. Describe guidelines for assisting with grooming

Multiple Choice.

Circle the letter of the answer that best completes the statement or answers the question.

1. Which of the following statements is true of nail care?

    a. NAs can use the same nail care equipment on more than one resident.

    b. A resident's routine and preferences for nail care are unimportant.

    c. NAs need to know what care to provide.

    d. NAs should clip a resident's toenails if they are getting long.

2. Which of the following statements is true of residents' toenails?

    a. NAs should never cut a resident's toenails.

    b. Diabetes has no effect on toenail care.

    c. NAs can clip a resident's toenails if he or she asks the NA to do it.

    d. The care plan does not need to be followed with regards to toenail care.

3. Which of the following does NOT help promote independence and dignity while assisting with grooming?

    a. You should do care for residents if you can do it faster than they can.

    b. You should allow residents to do all they can for themselves.

    c. You should let residents make as many choices as possible.

    d. You should follow residents' personal routines or particular ways of grooming themselves.

4. Which of the following is true of hair and hair care?

    a. Hair thickens as people age.

    b. Style residents' hair in childish styles.

    c. Handle hair very gently.

    d. It is okay to use the same comb and brush on different residents.

5. All of the following statements about pediculosis are true, EXCEPT:

    a. Special lice cream or shampoo may be used to treat lice.

    b. Symptoms of pediculosis include bite marks on the scalp, skin sores, and bad-smelling hair.

    c. Lice can spread very quickly and signs of lice must be reported immediately.

    d. If you think a resident does not have pediculosis, you can share combs, brushes, and wigs.

6. Briefly describe each razor.

A **safety** razor _____

_____

_____

_____

An **electric** razor _____

_____

_____

A **disposable** razor_____

_____

_____

_____

Unit 4. Identify guidelines for good oral hygiene

Crossword.

Clues:

Across

2. Breath that smells bad or like this must be reported

_____

5. Artificial teeth

_____

7. Flossing the teeth removes tartar and this

_____

9. When providing oral care you must wear these

_____

Down

1. With unconscious residents, it is impor-tant to use this as little as possible when performing mouth care.

_____

3. Oral care needs to include brushing this too, along with the teeth.

_____

4. The inhalation of food or drink into the lungs

_____

6. How often oral care is performed, at least, per day

_____

8. Canker sores or small, painful, white sores are examples of these, and they must be reported.

_____

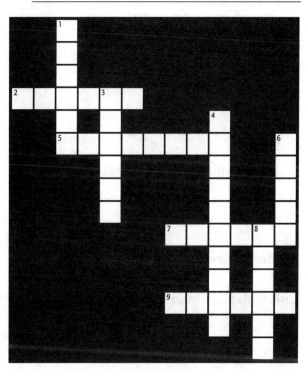

Unit 5. List guidelines for assisting with dressing

Fill in the Blank.

1. If a resident has a weakened side from a stroke or injury, that side is called the _____ side.

Name: _____

2. Use the terms _____ or _____ to refer to the affected side.

3. The _____ arm is usually placed through a sleeve first.

4. Encourage a resident to dress in _____ clothes rather than nightclothes.

5. Encourage and allow a resident to _____ clothing for the day.

6. Place the weak arm or leg through the garment first, then the _____ arm.

7. Having residents choose the clothes they will wear encourages

    _____ and promotes self-care.

8. IV stands for

    _____,

    or into a vein.

9. Always keep an IV bag

    _____ the IV site on body.

10. Remove or assist in removing clothing from the side

    _____ the IV first.

Unit 6. Explain guidelines for assisting with toileting

Matching.

Write the letter of the correct definition beside each term listed at right.

a. A bedpan that is flatter than the regular bedpan

b. Generally used by men for urination

c. A specific amount of water flowed into the colon to eliminate stool

d. An inability to control the muscles of the bowels or bladder

e. A chair with a toilet seat and a removable container underneath

f. A medication given rectally to cause a bowel movement

g. Difficult and often painful elimination of a hard, dry stool

h. A hard stool stuck in the rectum that cannot be expelled

1. _____ Constipation

2. _____ Portable commode

3. _____ Fracture pan

4. _____ Enema

5. _____ Urinal

6. _____ Fecal impaction

7. _____ Suppository

8. _____ Incontinence

Labeling.

Identify the following elimination supplies.

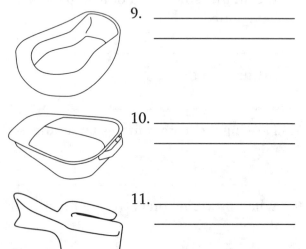

9. _____
   _____

10. _____
    _____

11. _____
    _____

Short Answer.

12. Why should a nursing assistant note the color, odor, and qualities of urine and

stool after a resident uses a bedpan, urinal, or commode?

_____

_____

_____

_____

_____

_____

_____

_____

4. _____

5. _____

6. _____

7. _____

8. _____

9. _____

10. _____

11. _____

12. _____

Unit 7. Identify guidelines for good skin care

Labeling.

Label the pressure sore danger areas. Some areas have already been filled in for you.

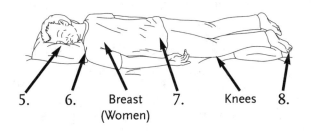

Side of Head 1. 2. 3. Greater Trochanter 4. Ankles

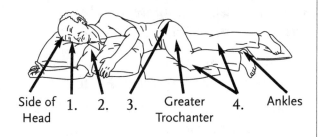

5. 6. Breast (Women) 7. Knees 8.

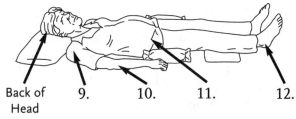

Back of Head 9. 10. 11. 12.

1. _____

2. _____

3. _____

Multiple Choice.

Circle the letter of the answer that best completes the statement or answers the question.

13. Which of the following increases the risk of pressure sores?

    a. Circulation

    b. Immobility

    c. Exercise

    d. Back rubs

14. Which of the following statements is true of pressure sores?

    a. Pressure sores are painful and difficult to heal. They can lead to life-threatening infection.

    b. Pressure sores cannot be prevented.

    c. Bony prominences are not at higher risk for pressure sores.

    d. Pulling residents across sheets during transfers will help prevent pressure sores.

15. Which stage of a pressure sore has the skin intact but showing redness that is not relieved within 15 to 30 minutes after removing pressure?

    a. Stage 1

    b. Stage 2

    c. Stage 3

    d. Stage 4

16. Which stage of a pressure sore has the ulcer looking like a deep crater, and full skin loss involving tissue damage that may extend down to, but not through, the tissue that covers muscle?

    a. Stage 1

    b. Stage 2

    c. Stage 3

    d. Stage 4

True or False.

Mark each statement with either a "T" for true or an "F" for false.

17. _____ Rashes or any discoloration of the skin are things you should report.

18. _____ You should reposition residents who cannot get out of bed at least every two hours.

19. _____ Pull residents across the sheets during transfers or repositioning.

20. _____ Back rubs can help relax residents and increase circulation.

21. _____ Residents seated in chairs or wheelchairs do not need to be repositioned.

22. _____ Sheepskin or bed pads absorb perspiration and protect the skin from irritating bed linens.

23. _____ Massage any white, red, or purple areas you see on a resident's skin.

Matching.

Write the letter of the correct definition beside each term listed at right.

a. Turning sheets placed under residents who cannot help with turning in bed, lifting, or moving up in bed

b. Keep the fingers from curling tightly

c. Used to keep the bed covers from pushing down on resident's feet

d. Padded boards placed against the resident's feet to keep them flexed

e. Used to keep joints in the correct position

24. _____ Bed cradles

25. _____ Footboards

26. _____ Hand rolls

27. _____ Splints

28. _____ Draw sheets

Unit 8. Explain the guidelines for safely positioning and transferring residents

Multiple Choice.

Circle the letter of the answer that best completes the statement or answers the question.

1. All of the following statements are true of positioning a resident, EXCEPT:

    a. When positioning residents, check the skin for signs of irritation.

    b. Bedbound residents should be repositioned every four hours.

    c. Positioning means helping residents into positions that are healthy and comfortable.

    d. Follow the care plan with regards to what kind of positioning you should do.

2. The practice of moving a resident as a unit, without disturbing the alignment of the body, is called:

    a. Dangling

    b. Ergonomics

    c. Logrolling

    d. Positioning

Name: _____

3. To minimize the manual lifting of residents, you should:

   a. Use the provided equipment properly

   b. Work by yourself to transfer or reposition residents

   c. Bend at the waist while lifting

   d. Never transfer residents

4. When a resident falls:

   a. Widen your stance and bring the resident's body close to you

   b. Catch the resident under the arms to stop the fall

   c. Try to reverse the fall

   d. Get the resident up after the fall

5. Which of the following statements about wheelchairs is NOT true?

   a. The wheelchair should be unlocked before assisting a resident into or out of it.

   b. You should know how to apply and release the brake and how to work the footrests.

   c. After a transfer, a wheelchair should be unlocked.

   d. Ask the resident how you can assist with wheelchairs. Some residents will want you to be more involved with the transfer.

6. When taking a resident down a ramp in a wheelchair, you should:

   a. Go forward, so the resident is facing the bottom of the ramp

   b. Go sideways, so the resident is facing the side of the ramp

   c. Find an alternate route and not use the ramp

   d. Go backwards, so the resident is facing the top of the ramp

7. A sliding board:

   a. May be used to help transfer residents who are unable to bear weight on their legs

   b. Should not be used for bed-to-chair transfers

   c. Fits around the resident's waist outside her clothing

   d. May only be used for residents who are able to bear weight on their legs

8. All of the following statements about transfer belts are true, EXCEPT:

   a. They are also called "gait belts" when helping a resident walk.

   b. They are applied underneath a resident's clothing.

   c. You need to leave enough room to insert four fingers into the belt.

   d. They are made of canvas or other heavy material.

Short Answer.

9. Why is it important to understand and use provided equipment when lifting or transferring a resident?

   _____
   _____
   _____
   _____
   _____
   _____

six

Basic Nursing Skills

Unit 1. Explain admission, transfer, and discharge of a resident

Word Search.

Complete each of the following sentences and find your answers in the word search.

r	l	q	s	n	o	i	t	s	e	u	q	r	k
u	j	l	t	u	t	y	y	m	x	c	u	m	g
m	v	r	x	i	m	f	d	w	a	s	w	a	d
j	f	f	x	s	m	q	o	r	h	y	o	g	m
e	u	l	l	r	h	p	e	r	w	z	c	g	s
v	k	q	j	o	t	f	r	t	m	d	d	i	v
c	o	c	n	k	u	p	m	e	s	a	n	j	o
i	n	i	n	l	r	o	n	e	s	u	l	j	y
h	o	p	l	e	e	s	j	p	a	s	j	x	e
g	f	y	p	g	b	s	j	j	d	q	i	d	f
m	z	a	n	n	h	o	l	t	k	h	w	o	a
x	r	a	x	n	w	e	l	q	u	g	e	c	n
e	h	p	o	s	i	t	i	v	e	d	d	e	d
c	h	e	k	x	e	c	u	d	o	r	t	n	i

1. Moving into a nursing home is a big
   _____.

2. Make sure a resident has a good
   _____
   of you and your facility.

3. Answer any _____
   a new resident has.

4. Never _____
   the process or the new resident.

5. Handle personal items
   _____
   and respectfully.

6. _____
   the resident to everyone you see.

7. _____
   the room before the resident arrives.

8. Always address the person with his
   _____
   name until he tells you what he wants to
   be called.

9. To lessen the stress of a transfer, inform
   the resident as soon as possible so he
   can begin to
   _____
   to the idea.

10. For a resident who is being discharged,
    be _____.
    Assure the resident he is ready for this
    important change.

Short Answer.

11. Why do you think it's important to make
    a new resident feel comfortable?

    _____
    _____
    _____
    _____
    _____
    _____
    _____
    _____
    _____

44

Unit 2. Explain the importance of monitoring vital signs

Short Answer.

What are the five vital signs that you will monitor?

1. _____

_____

2. _____

_____

3. _____

_____

4. _____

_____

5. _____

_____

Watching for changes in vital signs is important. What changes in vital signs need to be reported to the nurse right away?

6. _____

_____

_____

7. _____

_____

_____

8. _____

_____

_____

9. _____

_____

_____

The four sites for taking body temperature are:

10. _____

11. _____

12. _____

13. _____

List the normal ranges for vital signs.

Temperature: Fahrenheit   Celsius

14. Oral_____

15. Rectal _____

16. Axillary _____

17. Pulse_____

18. Respirations_____

_____

19. Blood Pressure_____

_____

20. What is generally considered to be the most accurate temperature site?

_____

_____

Write the temperature reading to the nearest tenth degree for each of the examples below.

21. _____

22. _____

23. _____

96   98 .6   100   2   4   6 °F
36   37   38   39   40   41 °C

24. _____

96   98 .6   100   2   4   6 °F
36   37   38   39   40   41 °C

25. _____

96   98 .6   100   2   4   6 °F
36   37   38   39   40   41 °C

26. _____

96   98 .6   100   2   4   6 °F
36   37   38   39   40   41 °C

27. _____

96   98 .6   100   2   4   6 °F
36   37   38   39   40   41 °C

28. _____

29. Why should you record vital signs immediately after taking them?

_____

_____

_____

_____

_____

30. Why should you count respirations immediately after taking the pulse?

_____

_____

Matching.

Write the letter of the correct definition beside each term listed below.

a. Brachial pulse

b. Respiration

c. Radial pulse

d. Inspiration

e. Diastolic

f. Expiration

g. Systolic

h. Hypertension

31. _____ A measurement of blood pressure showing when the heart is at work, contracting and pushing blood out of the left ventricle

32. _____ The process of breathing air into the lungs and exhaling air out of the lungs

33. _____ High blood pressure

34. _____ The most common site for checking the pulse, located on the inside of the wrist, where the radial artery runs just beneath the skin

35. _____ A measurement of blood pressure showing when the heart relaxes

36. _____ The pulse inside the elbow, about 1–1½ inches above the elbow

37. _____ Breathing air into the lungs

38. _____ Exhaling air out of the lungs

Multiple Choice.

Circle the letter of the answer that best completes the statement or answers the question.

39. Which of the following statements about pain is true?

   a. Pain is the same for everybody.

   b. Pain is a normal part of aging.

   c. Sustained pain may lead to withdrawal and depression.

   d. Do not take residents' complaints of pain seriously if they mention it often.

40. If a resident tells you she is in pain, how should you respond?

   a. Ask her questions about the pain, including where the pain is and when it started.

   b. Wait to report it to the nurse until you are sure the pain is serious.

   c. Take no action if the resident has already been given pain medication.

   d. Tell the resident that pain is a normal part of getting older and that she will have to adjust to it.

41. Which of the following may be a sign that a resident is in pain and should be reported?

   a. Laughing

   b. Squeezing eyes shut

   c. Smiling

   d. Eating

42. All of the following are ways to reduce pain, EXCEPT:

   a. Be patient and caring.

   b. Give back rubs.

   c. Provide a loud environment.

   d. Position the body in good alignment.

Unit 3. Explain how to measure height and weight

True or False.

Mark each statement with either a "T" for true or an "F" for false.

1. _____ If a resident loses one pound, you do not need to report it.

2. _____ On some wheelchair scales, you will need to subtract the weight of the wheelchair before recording a resident's weight.

3. _____ If a resident is unable to get out of bed, a special scale can be used to weigh him or her.

4. _____ Residents who are unable to get out of bed cannot have their height measured.

5. _____ For a resident who is bed-bound, measure height by marking on the sheet at the top of the head and at the bottom of the feet.

6. _____ You can measure the height of a resident who has contractures.

Labeling.

Looking at each of the scales below, how much does each resident weigh?

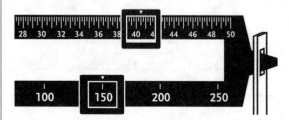

7. _____

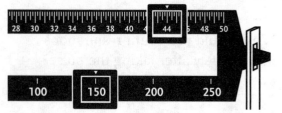

8. _____

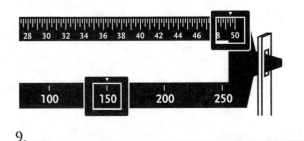

9. _____

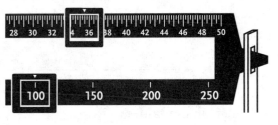

10. _____

Unit 4. Explain restraints and how to promote a restraint-free environment

Multiple Choice.

Circle the letter of the answer that best completes the statement or answers the question.

1. A restraint is a physical or chemical way to restrict movement or behavior. All of the following are examples of restraints, EXCEPT:

   a. Tying a resident's legs and arms to the bed

   b. Putting both side rails up on the bed

   c. Giving a resident medication to calm him down

   d. Giving a resident a repetitive task to do

2. Which of the following statements is true of restraints?

   a. Restraints can be used when staff is too busy to watch a resident.

   b. Restraints can cause incontinence, pressure sores, and even death.

   c. Restraints can be applied when a resident has said something mean to a nursing assistant.

   d. Restraint-free care means restraints are used only once a month.

3. Restraints can be applied:

   a. As punishment from staff when a resident isn't behaving properly

   b. When the nursing assistant feels like applying them

   c. Only with a doctor's order

   d. When a staff member doesn't have time to watch a resident closely

4. An example of a restraint alternative is:

   a. Not helping with toileting

   b. Stopping all exercise for a resident

   c. Answering a call light promptly

   d. Eliminating visits and social interaction

Short Answer.

5. When a resident is restrained, he or she has to be monitored continuously. The resident must be checked at least every 15 minutes. What needs to happen at least every two hours, or as needed?

   _____

   _____

   _____

   _____

   _____

   _____

   _____

   _____

6. How do you think you would feel if you were restrained? Can you understand why it might make someone feel a loss of dignity or feel depressed?

   _____

   _____

   _____

   _____

Name: _____

Unit 5. Define fluid balance and explain intake and output (I&O)

Fill in the Blank.

1. _____
   is maintaining equal intake and output of fluids.

2. The fluid a person consumes is called _____.

3. _____ is eliminated fluid; it includes urine, feces, and vomitus.

4. A _____ is a tube used to drain urine from the bladder.

5. A catheter drainage bag must always be kept _____ than the hips or bladder.

6. Catheter tubing should be kept as _____ as possible and should not be _____.

7. An indwelling catheter remains inside the _____ for a period of time.

8. A _____ catheter has an attachment on the end that fits onto the penis.

9. _____ and _____ are two types of specimens you may be asked to collect from a resident.

10. _____ is mucus coughed up from the lungs.

11. A _____ urine specimen does not include the first and last urine in the sample.

12. When cleaning catheter tubing, clean at least _____ inches of it nearest meatus. Move in

only one direction, _____ from meatus. Use a _____ area of the cloth for each stroke.

Short Answer.

13. How many cubic centimeters (cc) equal 1 ounce (oz.)?

_____

List the amount of fluid in cubic centimeters (cc) in each container.

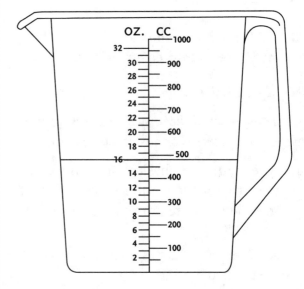

14. _____

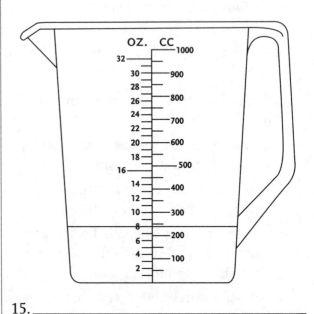

15. _____

Name: _____

Unit 6. Explain care guidelines for different types of tubing

Mark an "X" by all of the correct guidelines for working around oxygen equipment.

1. _____ It is okay to smoke in a room where oxygen is used or stored.

2. _____ Remove all fire hazards from the room or area if oxygen is present.

3. _____ Fire hazards can be electric shavers, hair dryers, or other electrical appliances.

4. _____ Nursing assistants can adjust oxygen levels.

5. _____ Never allow candles or other open flames around oxygen.

6. _____ Check behind the ears for irritation from nasal cannula.

7. _____ Oxygen can come in tanks or an oxygen concentrator.

Short Answer.

8. List eight items to report about an IV.

_____

_____

_____

_____

_____

_____

_____

_____

_____

_____

_____

Unit 7. Discuss a resident's unit and related care

Fill in the Blank.

1. The resident's unit is the resident's home and must be treated with

_____.

2. Knock and wait for

_____

before entering a resident's room.

3. Bedside stands can store

_____

items.

4. The _____
table may be used for meals or personal care; it is a clean area.

5. Do not place

_____

and urinals on the overbed table.

6. Answer call lights

_____.

7. Keep call lights within residents'

_____.

8. Refill _____
pitchers regularly unless the resident has a fluid restriction.

9. Re-stock _____
before leaving a resident's room; they include tissue, paper towels, soap, or any other needed items.

10. If you find

_____

equipment, such as frayed or cracked cords, report it to the nurse.

11. Clean up _____
promptly.

12. Do not move residents'

_____.

Name: _____

Unit 8. Explain the importance of sleep and perform proper bedmaking

Crossword.

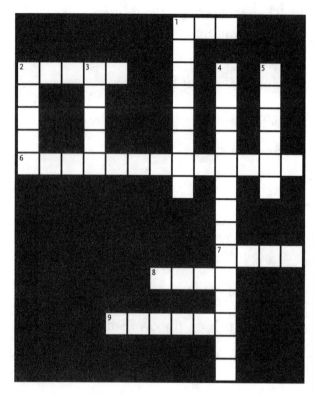

Clues:

Across

1. Change linens when soiled, wrinkled, or this.

   _____

2. Do not do this to linen, as it may spread airborne contaminants.

   _____

6. Residents who spend long hours in bed are at risk for these.

   _____

7. You carry bed linen _____ from your uniform.

8. Turn a closed bed into this by folding the linen down to the foot of the bed.

   _____

9. Wear these when removing bed linens.

   _____

Down

1. Keep beds smooth and free of crumbs and these.

   _____

2. Provides the body with new cells and energy

   _____

3. You don't bend at the waist to make a bed; you bend these.

   _____

4. These thrive in moist, warm environments.

   _____

5. A bed completely made with the bed-spread and blankets in place

   _____

Unit 9. Explain how to apply non-sterile dressings

Fill in the Blank.

1. Sterile dressings are those that cover _____ or _____ wounds. A _____ always changes these dressings. Non-sterile dressings are applied to _____ wounds that have less chance of

   _____.

seven

Nutrition and Hydration

Unit 1. Identify the six basic nutrients and explain MyPyramid

Read the following sentences and mark which of the six basic nutrients each is describing. Use a "P" for proteins, "C" for carbohydrates, "F" for fats, "V" for vitamins, "M" for minerals, and "W" for water.

1. _____ Good sources of these are fish, meat, dried beans, and cheese.

2. _____ Without this, a person can only live for a few days.

3. _____ These help the body store energy.

4. _____ It protects organs and helps the body absorb certain vitamins.

5. _____ Beans and rice are examples of complementary _____.

6. _____ Examples of these are butter, oil, and salad dressing.

7. _____ They are essential for tissue growth and repair.

8. _____ Most of these cannot be produced by the body.

9. _____ Simple _____ are stored as fat.

10. _____ Examples of these include bread, cereal, and potatoes.

11. _____ This is the most essential nutrient for life.

12. _____ Through perspiration, this helps to maintain body temperature.

13. _____ These can be fat-soluble or water-soluble.

14. _____ One-half to two-thirds of our body weight is this.

15. _____ Iron and calcium are examples of these.

Labeling.

Looking at MyPyramid below, fill in the six food groups and one additional element of good health.

16. _____

17. _____

18. _____

19. _____

20. _____

21. _____

22. _____

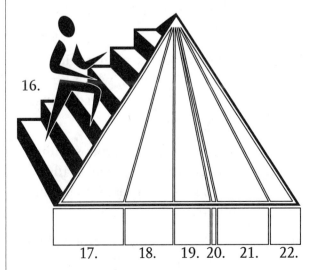

16.

17.   18.   19. 20. 21.   22.

Read the following descriptions and mark which each is describing—"G" for grains, "FR" for fruits, "V" for vegetables, "M" for milk products, "MB" for meats and beans, "O" for oils, "A" for activity.

23. _____ This group includes foods that retain their calcium content, such as yogurt and cheese.

24. _____ Includes all foods made from wheat, rice, oats, cornmeal, and barley.

25. _____ Foods that are mainly this include mayonnaise, some salad dressings, and soft margarine.

26. _____ One ounce of lean poultry, one egg, or 1/2 ounce of nuts or seeds can be considered as one ounce equivalent from this group.

27. _____ This should be done for at least 30 minutes per day.

28. _____ Important sources of dietary fiber and many nutrients, including folic acid and Vitamin C.

29. _____ Most of these eaten should be polyunstaurated (PUFA).

30. _____ At least half of all of these consumed should be "whole."

31. _____ This increases the amount of calories burned.

32. _____ These products are the primary source of calcium, which builds bones and teeth and maintains bone mass.

33. _____ There are five subgroups within this group: dark green, orange, dry beans and peas, starchy, and others.

34. _____ Most choices in this group should be lean or low-fat.

Unit 2. Demonstrate an awareness of regional, cultural, and religious food preferences

Short Answer.

Briefly describe some of the foods you ate while growing up. Were there any special dishes that your family made that were related to your culture, religion, or region?

_____

_____

_____

_____

_____

_____

Unit 3. Explain special diets

Matching.

Read the following sentences and identify what special diet each is describing. Choose from the diets listed below.

a. Low-sodium diet
b. Fluid-restricted diet
c. Low-protein diet
d. Low-fat/Low-cholesterol diet
e. Modified calorie diet
f. Dietary management of diabetes
g. Liquid diet
h. Soft diet
i. Pureed diet
j. NPO

1. _____ To prevent further heart or kidney damage, doctors may restrict a resident's fluid intake.

2. _____ People who have kidney disease may also be on this diet.

3. _____ People at risk for heart attacks and heart disease may be placed on these. This diet permits skim milk and low-fat meats and cheese.

4. _____ Calories and carbohydrates must be carefully controlled in this diet. The types and amounts of foods are determined by nutritional and energy needs.

5. _____ This diet consists of foods that are in a liquid state at body temperature.

6. _____ Salt is restricted in this diet. Abbreviations for this diet are "Low Na" and "NAS."

7. _____ This abbreviation means that a person is not allowed to have anything to eat or drink by mouth.

8. _____ This diet consists of soft or chopped foods that are easy to chew and swallow.

9. _____ Used for losing weight or preventing additional weight gain.

10. _____ This diet consists of foods thick enough to hold their form in the mouth; this diet does not require a person to chew his food.

Unit 4. Understand the importance of observing and reporting a resident's diet

Short Answer.

1. List three things you must make sure of before delivering trays or plates.

_____

_____

_____

_____

_____

_____

_____

_____

_____

2. What are two reasons you should observe what a resident eats?

_____

_____

_____

_____

_____

_____

_____

_____

Unit 5. Describe how to assist residents in maintaining fluid balance

Fill in the Blank.

1. The sense of _____ can lessen as people age.

2. Most residents should be encouraged to drink at least _____ glasses of water or other fluids a day.

3. _____ is an order that means to encourage the person to drink more fluids.

4. _____ occurs when a person does not have enough fluid in the body.

5. Encourage residents to

_____

every time you see them.

6. Offer fresh _____ or other fluids often.

Name: _____

7. _____
is an order that means the person is allowed to drink, but must limit the daily amount to a level set by the doctor.

8. _____
is swelling caused by excess fluid in the body.

9. Make sure pitcher and cup are near enough and _____ enough for the resident to lift.

10. If appropriate, offer sips of liquid _____ bites of food at meals and snacks.

11. _____
occurs when the body is unable to handle the amount of fluid consumed.

Short Answer.

12. List ten things to observe and report about dehydration.

_____

_____

_____

_____

_____

_____

_____

_____

_____

_____

_____

_____

_____

_____

13. List six things to observe and report about fluid overload.

_____

_____

_____

_____

_____

_____

_____

_____

_____

_____

Unit 6. List ways to identify and prevent unintended weight loss

Word Search.

Complete each of the following sentences and find your answers in the word search.

e	u	a	x	w	e	r	a	c	l	a	r	o	u
e	k	j	i	l	n	s	t	u	m	b	b	p	s
j	e	a	e	j	e	t	s	w	y	e	r	y	e
l	r	t	t	p	s	f	l	v	v	i	g	z	c
q	c	x	i	n	z	k	n	e	g	p	a	p	d
l	j	o	f	t	i	g	r	h	p	y	e	p	o
i	v	p	i	c	e	a	t	u	e	s	v	b	h
b	w	m	v	m	g	p	c	m	d	v	a	a	x
j	n	o	u	e	j	z	p	l	u	j	q	l	m
d	o	q	s	w	f	z	l	a	o	b	w	m	w
t	a	t	d	b	n	t	o	x	m	e	c	l	p
c	a	o	o	u	d	x	g	e	k	d	m	z	n
e	o	w	i	x	v	a	g	c	c	d	c	i	u
f	u	t	e	n	s	i	l	s	i	i	w	c	t

1. Encourage residents to _____.

2. Give _____ before and after meals.

3. Honor residents'
    _____ likes
    and dislikes.

4. Offer many different kinds of foods and
    _____.

5. Allow enough _____
    to finish eating.

6. Notify nurse if resident has trouble
    using _____.

7. Position residents sitting
    _____ for feeding.

8. If resident has had a loss of
    _____,
    ask about it.

9. Record meal/snack
    _____.

Unit 7. Identify ways to promote appetites at mealtime

Case Study.

Read the following paragraph and answer the question.

Susana, a nursing assistant, enters Mr. Franti's room to assist him with his dinner. She tells him hello and asks him if he would like to wear a clothing protector while dining. He says yes. She puts on the protector and brings the tray over. She cuts his food into small pieces and notices that his meat is almost cold. She offers him a fork. He can't grasp it so she begins feeding him herself. She stares out the window while offering him bites of food. He says that he is finished. She looks down and notices that he has barely touched his food.

1. What are some ways that Susana could have better promoted her resident's appetite? What important things did she forget? What did she do right?

_____

_____

_____

_____

_____

_____

_____

_____

_____

_____

_____

_____

_____

_____

_____

_____

_____

Short Answer.

2. If a resident is eating in the dining room and has poor sitting balance, how can you help?

_____

_____

_____

_____

_____

_____

_____

_____

_____

Name: _____

Unit 8. Demonstrate ways to feed residents

Multiple Choice.

Circle the letter of the answer that best completes the statement or answers the question.

1. When assisting residents with eating, a nursing assistant should:

   a. Verify that she has the right resident by checking the diet card against the resident's identification

   b. Rush the resident through his meal

   c. Mix all of the resident's foods together

   d. Blow on hot food to cool it off

2. Ways to promote a resident's dignity while feeding include:

   a. Telling him, "Hurry up. I've got three other people to feed."

   b. Asking him, "What would you like to try first?"

   c. Looking around the room while he is eating

   d. Doing everything for him, even if he can do tasks himself

3. How should you test the temperature of food?

   a. Touch it with your fingers

   b. Blow on it first, then touch it

   c. Put your hand over the dish to sense the heat

   d. Eat some of the food to test it

4. A resident who has had a stroke may benefit from:

   a. The NA doing everything for the resident

   b. Physical cues

   c. No help from the NA

   d. The NA not identifying the resident before feeding

True or False.

Mark each statement with either a "T" for true or an "F" for false.

5. _____ If a resident says, "I don't want to wear a clothing protector," you should put one on her anyway.

6. _____ Residents who must be fed are often embarrassed and depressed about their dependence on another person.

7. _____ Some residents will only need help with setting up. Once that is done, the NA will only need to check in with them from time to time.

8. _____ If a resident can use and hold a napkin, she should.

9. _____ It is not necessary to identify residents before feeding them.

10. _____ Identify foods, even pureed foods, by their correct names.

11. _____ Alternate food and drink while feeding.

12. _____ Remain completely silent while feeding residents.

13. _____ Sit higher than a resident while feeding.

14. _____ You should give a resident your full attention during eating.

15. _____ Residents have the right to ask for and receive different food.

16. _____ When feeding a resident, make sure the resident's mouth is empty before giving another bite of food or sip of beverage.

17. _____ You will choose which food a resident eats first, not the resident.

18. _____ A resident should be fed lying flat on his back.

19. _____ Adaptive devices can help residents eat.

20. _____ Mix all the residents' foods together without asking him about this.

Unit 9. Describe eating and swallowing problems a resident may have

Fill in the Blank.

1. _____ is difficulty swallowing.

2. Conditions that may make eating and swallowing difficult are

_____,

cancer, Multiple Sclerosis, Parkinson's, or Alzheimer's disease.

3. _____

improves the ability to control fluid in the mouth and throat.

4. The consistency that is the thickness of a thick juice, such as pear nectar or tomato is called

_____ thick.

5. The consistency that has the thickness of honey is called

_____ thick.

6. The consistency in which liquids have become semi-solid and must be consumed with a spoon is called

_____ thick.

7. _____ is the inhalation of food or drink into the lungs.

8. A tube that is inserted into the nose and goes into the stomach to feed residents is called a

_____ tube.

9. A tube that is placed through the skin directly into the stomach is called a

_____ tube.

10. If a person's digestive system does not function properly, hyperalimentation or

_____

may be needed.

Short Answer.

Mark an "X" by all of the correct guidelines for working with residents with tube feedings.

11. _____ Make sure that tubing is kinked.

12. _____ Only doctors or nurses insert or remove tubes.

13. _____ During the feeding, the resident should remain in a sitting position with the head of the bed elevated about 45 degrees.

14. _____ Provide frequent mouth and nose care.

15. _____ Keep resident on top of the tubing.

16. _____ Nursing assistants perform tube feedings.

17. _____ Watch for signs of infection, including redness or drainage around the opening.

18. _____ Nursing assistants clean the tubing.

19. List ten signs and symptoms of swallowing problems that must be reported.

_____
_____
_____
_____
_____
_____
_____
_____
_____
_____

Name: _____

_____

_____

_____

_____

20. List five ways to prevent aspiration.

_____

_____

_____

_____

_____

_____

_____

_____

_____

Unit 10. Describe how to assist residents with special needs

Word Search.

Complete each of the following sentences and find your answers in the word search.

e	l	r	p	w	l	d	q	w	v	a	d	x	i
f	s	u	h	e	k	a	l	t	s	c	k	a	o
j	i	i	e	r	s	x	m	s	e	v	c	d	a
s	y	e	x	t	v	z	i	r	v	a	o	u	z
p	u	x	l	n	z	s	c	v	o	e	l	n	v
k	p	c	u	d	t	p	b	x	z	n	c	a	d
l	f	w	l	i	o	w	b	g	w	y	x	f	s
p	s	x	v	b	x	f	s	o	f	t	z	f	a
i	q	e	p	x	q	c	v	i	q	s	y	e	r
b	s	r	o	m	e	r	t	i	k	o	e	c	v
k	l	u	d	m	p	d	p	x	s	z	a	t	v
v	s	a	u	z	z	m	x	j	v	i	a	e	h
s	e	n	a	k	f	v	a	n	o	v	o	d	d
r	g	q	g	b	e	c	o	m	b	f	b	n	q

1. For visually-impaired residents, use the face of an imaginary _____

to explain the positions of objects in front of them.

2. Always place food in the _____, or non-paralyzed, side of the mouth.

3. _____ or shaking make it difficult for a person with Parkinson's disease to eat.

4. _____ devices make it easier for a resident to eat and promote independence.

5. Face visually-impaired residents when speaking and use a _____ tone of voice.

6. For residents who have had a stroke, food must be placed in their _____, which is determined by a nurse.

7. At mealtime, _____ the menu to a visually-impaired resident.

8. For residents who have had a stroke, serve _____ foods if swallowing is difficult.

eight

Common, Chronic, and Acute Conditions

Unit 1. Describe common diseases and disorders of the musculoskeletal system

Multiple Choice.

Circle the correct response.

1. Which of the following terms means an illness or long-term?
   a. Acute
   b. Chronic
   c. Inflammation
   d. Menopause

2. _____ is a common type of arthritis in which weight-bearing joints, such as the hips and knees, are affected.
   a. Osteoarthritis
   b. Autoimmune
   c. Osteoporosis
   d. Acute

3. Treatment for arthritis includes:
   a. Doing no activity whatsoever
   b. Assuming each resident has the same symptoms
   c. Adding extra calories into the diet to help the resident gain weight
   d. Taking anti-inflammatory medications, such as aspirin or ibuprofen

4. All of the following are care guidelines for arthritis, EXCEPT:
   a. Do not promote independence by offering special devices.
   b. Choose clothing that is easy to put on.
   c. Have a positive attitude.
   d. Treat each resident as an individual.

Fill in the Blank.

5. _____ is the stopping of menstrual periods.

6. Brittle bones are bones that can _____ easily.

7. Extra calcium and regular _____ can help prevent osteoporosis.

8. _____, calcium, and _____ are used to treat osteoporosis.

9. Nursing assistants must _____ residents with osteoporosis very carefully.

10. A broken bone is called a _____.

11. Preventing _____, which can lead to fractures, is very important.

12. After hip replacement surgery, a person is not able to _____ on that leg while the hip heals.

Word Search.

Look at the care guidelines for hip replacement. Complete each of the following sentences and find your answers in the word search.

13. Keep often-used items within easy _____.

14. Dress starting with the _____ side first.

Name: _____

15. Never _____
the resident. Use praise and encouragement.

16. Have the resident sit to do tasks and save _____.

17. Caution the resident not to

_____

legs or turn toes inward.

18. Being able to support some weight on one or both legs is called

_____

weight bearing.

Report these signs to the nurse:

19. If incision is _____,
draining, bleeding, or

_____ to touch

20. An increase in _____

21. Abnormal _____,
especially elevated temperature

22. Following doctor's orders for activity and

_____

23. Numbness or

_____

t	c	l	m	q	e	h	f	s	p	z	v	o	j
h	i	r	w	n	x	s	j	n	a	m	w	c	g
l	a	n	e	e	v	u	l	g	r	f	n	k	c
w	s	r	g	a	v	r	q	i	t	j	t	f	o
f	g	s	n	l	k	x	y	s	i	j	y	h	x
y	k	h	o	c	i	g	f	l	a	o	k	e	i
a	c	f	b	r	k	n	d	a	l	k	a	q	w
p	c	o	u	y	c	e	g	t	b	c	g	u	z
p	a	i	n	r	t	b	k	i	g	z	c	i	s
g	u	z	u	c	e	b	j	v	m	s	f	n	r
p	q	k	e	u	e	d	j	b	o	v	p	y	m
t	c	f	s	f	j	y	m	o	b	f	w	e	e
h	f	u	d	c	e	h	i	v	f	l	d	s	x
a	e	x	e	r	c	i	s	e	h	c	a	e	r

Short Answer.

Looking at the two illustrations below, which one is showing a 90-degree angle? A person recovering from hip replacement cannot bend the hip at an angle greater than this.

a.   b.

24. _____

True or False.

Mark each statement with either a "T" for true or an "F" for false.

25. _____ Recovery time for a knee replacement is usually much longer than for a hip replacement.

26. _____ Anti-embolic stockings aid circulation.

27. _____ Fluids high in Vitamin C can help prevent UTIs.

28. _____ Pain medications, if needed, are best given after moving and positioning residents.

29. _____ A compression stocking is hooked up to a machine that inflates and deflates on its own to mimic muscle movement.

Unit 2. Describe common diseases and disorders of the nervous system

True or False.

Mark each statement with either a "T" for true or an "F" for false.

1. _____ Confusion interferes with the ability to make decisions and personality may change.

2. _____ Confusion is always permanent.

3. _____ It is okay to leave a confused resident by himself.

4. _____ When talking to a confused resident, speak clearly and slowly in a lower tone of voice.

5. _____ Do not tell confused residents what the plans for the day are.

Short Answer.

For each of the following guidelines for working with residents with Alzheimer's disease, briefly describe why you think this guideline is helpful.

6. Do not take their behavior personally. Why?

_____
_____
_____
_____
_____
_____
_____
_____
_____

7. Treat them with dignity and respect. Why?

_____
_____
_____
_____
_____
_____
_____
_____

8. Work with the symptoms and behaviors you see. Why?

_____
_____
_____
_____
_____
_____
_____
_____

9. Work as a team. Why?

_____
_____
_____
_____
_____
_____
_____

10. Encourage communication. Why?

_____
_____
_____
_____
_____
_____

11. Take care of yourself. Why?

_____
_____
_____

Name: _____

_____
_____
_____
_____
_____

12. Work with family members. Why?

_____
_____
_____
_____
_____
_____
_____

13. Follow the goals of the resident care plan. Why?

_____
_____
_____
_____
_____
_____
_____
_____

True or False.

Mark each statement with either a "T" for true or an "F" for false.

14. _____ When communicating with an Alzheimer's resident, speak in a low, calm voice.

15. _____ Plenty of noise and distractions can help the resident cope with having Alzheimer's disease.

16. _____ When working with an Alzheimer's resident, you may have to repeat yourself several times.

17. _____ You should always use the same words and phrases when repeating something.

18. _____ A drawing of a toilet can be a form of communication.

19. _____ Dementia is a normal part of aging.

20. _____ Alzheimer's disease can be cured.

21. _____ Each person with AD will show different symptoms at different times.

22. _____ Encouraging residents with AD to perform ADLs and keep their minds and bodies as active as possible is important.

Short Answer.

For each of the guidelines for residents with Alzheimer's, write "yes" if the statement is correct, and "no" if the statement is incorrect.

23. _____ Use non-slip mats, tub seats, and hand-holds to ensure safety during bathing.

24. _____ Always bathe the resident at the same time every day, even if she is agitated.

25. _____ Always use the same steps and explain what you are doing the same way every time.

26. _____ Do not attempt to groom the resident, since people with AD cannot appreciate it.

27. _____ Mark the restroom with a sign as a reminder to use it.

28. _____ Do not encourage exercise. This will make the resident agitated.

29. _____ Do not encourage independence as this can lead to aggressive behavior.

30. _____ Share in enjoyable activities.

31. _____ Reward positive behavior with smiles, hugs, warm touches, and thank yous.

Multiple Choice.

Circle the correct response.

32. To help identify and remove triggers when a resident is agitated, the nursing assistant should:
    a. Keep a constant routine.
    b. Turn up the volume on the TV to soothe the resident.
    c. Change the routine constantly to keep the resident distracted.
    d. Speak in a loud voice.

33. How can a nursing assistant best respond to pacing and wandering?
    a. Keep the resident from moving and exercising.
    b. Suggest another activity.
    c. Eliminate snacks.
    d. Restrain the resident.

34. If a resident with AD is having delusions, the nursing assistant should:
    a. Tell the resident that what he believes is not true.
    b. Make a joke about the delusion to lighten the tension.
    c. Agree that the delusion is true.
    d. Calmly redirect the resident's interest.

35. The best response to sundowning is:
    a. Add caffeine into the diet.
    b. Change caregivers often.
    c. Plan social activities right before bed.
    d. Give a soothing massage.

36. When a person with AD overreacts to something in an unreasonable way, it is called:
    a. Perseveration
    b. Catastrophic reaction
    c. Hallucination
    d. Sundowning

37. When a resident perseverates, the nursing assistant should:
    a. Ask him to stop.
    b. Explain that what he is doing is perseverating.
    c. Answer question each time using the same words.
    d. Answer the question only once, as repeating answers will only encourage the behavior.

38. The most appropriate response to a violent resident is to:
    a. Step out of the resident's reach.
    b. Hit the resident back.
    c. Threaten the resident.
    d. Remain alone with the resident.

39. All of the following are good responses to disruptive behavior, EXCEPT:
    a. Encourage the resident to join in independent activities that are safe.
    b. Tactfully praise improvements in behavior.
    c. Do not involve resident in planning routines and schedules.
    d. Direct resident to a private area.

40. Which of the following statements is true of inappropriate sexual behavior?
    a. All sexual behavior from residents is intentional.
    b. It is okay to overreact to the behavior if it bothers you.
    c. Gently direct the resident to a private area and tell the nurse.
    d. Tell other residents what happened.

Name: _____

41. Which of the following statements is true of pillaging and hoarding?

  a. It is intentional behavior.

  b. Pillaging and hoarding should not be considered stealing.

  c. The resident knows what she is doing when she pillages.

  d. The nursing assistant should let the resident's family know that the resident is stealing from others.

Short Answer.

Choose which creative therapy for Alzheimer's disease is being described in each sentence.

  Activity Therapy
  Reality Orientation
  Reminiscence Therapy
  Validation Therapy

42. Encouraging the resident to talk about the past and explore memories.

  _____

43. Using calendars, clocks, signs, and lists to help the resident remember who and where she is.

  _____

44. Using activities to prevent boredom and frustration and improve self-esteem.

  _____

45. Letting the resident believe he lives in the past or in imaginary circumstances, without attempting to reorient him.

  _____

46. Asking a resident to tell you about where he was sent in the war and exploring details about his experiences.

  _____

Short Answer.

47. List five guidelines for caring for someone who has Parkinson's disease.

_____
_____
_____
_____
_____
_____

48. List eight guidelines for caring for someone who has Multiple Sclerosis.

_____
_____
_____
_____
_____
_____
_____
_____
_____
_____
_____

Scenarios.

Read each of the following statements, and answer the questions.

Kate, a nursing assistant, is getting ready to take Mr. Elliot, who is recovering from a stroke, on a walk. Mr. Elliot has difficulty communicating and suffers from confusion. "Let's see," Kate says. "We can walk to the gardens, the activity room, or the front area. Now, where would you like to go?"

49. What is wrong with the way Kate is communicating with Mr. Elliot?

_____
_____
_____
_____

Name: _____

_____
_____
_____
_____
_____

Kate notices that Mr. Elliot seems to be having trouble saying words clearly. He is beginning to get frustrated because he can't tell Kate what he wants. Kate decides to ask only "yes" or "no" questions, so she tells Mr. Elliot, "If you find it too difficult to speak right now, why don't you try nodding your head for 'yes' and shaking your head for 'no'."

50. What is Kate doing right?

_____
_____
_____
_____
_____
_____
_____
_____
_____
_____

Fill in the Blank.

51. When assisting with a transfer for a resident with one-sided weakness, always lead with the _____ side.

52. Dress the _____ side first. This prevents unnecessary _____ and _____ of the limb.

53. Undress the _____ side first.

54. _____ is used to help the resident dress himself.

True or False.

Mark each statement with either a "T" for true or an "F" for false.

55. _____ Residents with paralysis or loss of movement do not need physical therapy.

56. _____ Leg exercises improve circulation.

57. _____ When helping with transfers or ambulation, stand on the resident's stronger side.

58. _____ Always use a gait belt for safety.

59. _____ Refer to the side that has been affected by stroke as the "weaker" or "involved" side.

60. _____ Gestures and facial expressions are important in communicating with a resident who has had a stroke.

61. _____ Residents who suffer confusion or memory loss due to a stroke may feel more secure if you establish a routine of care.

62. _____ Residents may cry for no reason after suffering a stroke.

63. _____ Let the resident do things for him- or herself whenever possible.

64. _____ "Yes" or "no" questions are best to use with a resident who has had a stroke.

65. _____ Dress the stronger side first when assisting with dressing.

66

Name: _____

Short Answer.

66. Which illustration, the left or the right, shows a proper transfer of a resident with a one-sided weakness?

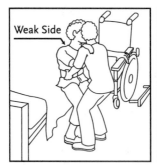 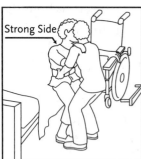

Weak Side   Strong Side

_____

67. List eight guidelines for caring for a person with a head or spinal cord injury.

_____

_____

_____

_____

_____

_____

_____

_____

_____

_____

_____

Unit 3. Describe common diseases and disorders of the circulatory system

Crossword.

Clues:

Across

2. The condition that occurs when blood flow to the heart muscle is completely blocked and the muscle cell dies

_____

4. PVD causes legs, feet, arms or hands to not have enough blood circulation. Skin may be pale or this color.

_____

8. Medication used to relax the walls of the coronary arteries.

_____

10. Drugs that reduce fluid in the body.

_____

Down

1. Elastic leg stockings, also called _____ hose, applied to reduce swelling in feet and ankles.

_____

3. The abbreviation for the condition of blood backing up into the heart instead of circulating

_____

5. Medications that remove fluids from the body may mean more trips to the bathroom. NAs must answer these requests promptly.

_____

6. Another name for high blood pressure

_____

7. Another name for chest pain

_____

9. With angina pectoris, this is very important. It reduces the heart's need for extra oxygen. It helps the blood flow return to normal, often within 3 to 15 minutes.

_____

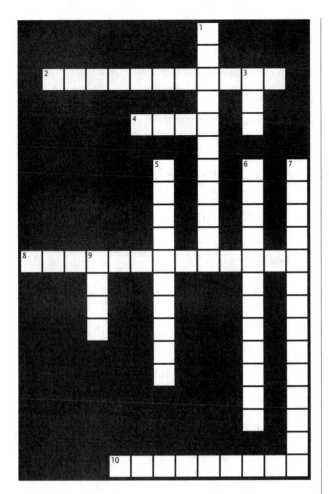

Unit 4. Describe common diseases and disorders of the respiratory system

Multiple Choice.

Circle the letter of the answer that best completes the statement or answers the question.

1. Residents with COPD have difficulty with this:
   a. Breathing
   b. Urination
   c. Weight
   d. Vision

2. A constant fear of a person who has COPD is:
   a. Constipation
   b. Incontinence
   c. Not being able to breathe
   d. Heart attack

3. Residents who have COPD can experience the following:
   a. Better appetites
   b. Extra sleep
   c. Fear of suffocation
   d. Ease of breathing

4. A resident with COPD should be positioned:
   a. Lying flat on his back
   b. Sitting upright
   c. Lying on his stomach
   d. Lying on his side

5. The NA's role in caring for a resident with COPD includes all of the following, EXCEPT:
   a. Being calm and supportive
   b. Encouraging independence
   c. Using good infection control
   d. Doing everything for the resident

Short Answer.

6. Which illustration, the left or the right, shows a more comfortable position for residents with COPD?

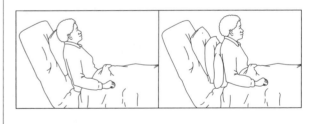

_____

_____

Unit 5. Describe common diseases and disorders of the urinary system

Fill in the Blank.

1. Females should always wipe from

_____ to

_____ after

elimination.

Name: _____

2. UTIs are more common in

   _____.

3. UTIs result in _____ during urination. They also cause a frequent feeling of needing to

   _____.

4. Encourage plenty of
   _____. Vitamin
   _____ helps acidify urine and prevent infection.

5. Offer a bedpan or a trip to the toilet at least every _____ hours. Answer call lights promptly.

6. Report _____, dark, or foul-smelling urine or if a resident urinates

   _____.

Unit 6. Describe common diseases and disorders of the gastrointestinal system

Multiple Choice.

Circle the letter of the answer that best completes the statement or answers the question.

1. An operation to create an opening from an area inside the body to the outside is:

   a. An ostomy

   b. A nasogastric tube

   c. A stoma

   d. GERD

2. Residents with ostomies may feel they have lost control of a basic bodily function. They may be embarrassed or angry about the ostomy. All of the following are good ideas for how an NA should respond, EXCEPT:

   a. By being sensitive

   b. By being supportive

   c. By providing privacy

   d. By rushing the resident

3. How often should an ostomy bag be emptied?

   a. Whenever a stool is eliminated

   b. Every 10 minutes

   c. Every 30 minutes

   d. Once a week

4. Which of the following is helpful for a resident who has GERD?

   a. Encourage spicy foods.

   b. Ask the resident not to lie down until at least two hours after eating.

   c. Serve the largest meal of the day at dinner.

   d. Keep the body lying flat during sleep.

Unit 7. Describe common diseases and disorders of the endocrine system

Short Answer.

1. List and briefly define the two major types of diabetes.

   _____

   _____

   _____

   _____

   _____

   _____

   _____

   _____

   _____

   _____

   _____

   _____

   _____

   _____

   _____

2. List eight symptoms that people with diabetes may have.

_____

_____

_____

_____

_____

_____

_____

_____

_____

3. Why must nursing assistants only perform foot care for diabetics as directed?

_____

_____

_____

_____

_____

4. List five important guidelines NAs can follow when caring for residents with diabetes.

_____

_____

_____

_____

_____

_____

_____

_____

_____

5. How much should a diabetic resident eat of food served?

_____

_____

Unit 8. Describe common diseases and disorders of the reproductive system

Fill in the Blank.

1. _____ is an infection of the vagina. Women who have this often have a _____ vaginal discharge. This is accompanied by _____ and burning.

2. With benign prostatic hypertrophy the prostate becomes

   _____.

   This causes pressure on the

   _____, which leads to problems

   _____ and/or emptying the bladder.

Unit 9. Describe common diseases and disorders of the immune and lymphatic systems

Multiple Choice.

Circle the letter of the answer that best completes the statement or answers the question.

1. Care for the person with AIDS should focus on:
   a. Helping to find a cure for AIDS
   b. Preventing transmission of AIDS to others
   c. Relieving symptoms and preventing infection
   d. Informing the resident's friends and family about his condition

2. How is HIV spread?
   a. By sex
   b. By handshakes
   c. By hugs
   d. By coughing

Name: _____

3. AIDS residents who have infections of the mouth may need to eat food that is:

   a. Spicy

   b. Soft

   c. Dry

   d. Very cold

4. Someone who has nausea and vomiting should:

   a. Eat small frequent meals

   b. Eat quickly

   c. Avoid drinking fluids

   d. Eat one big meal per day

5. The "BRAT" diet is helpful for:

   a. Diarrhea

   b. Weight gain

   c. Weight loss

   d. Numbness and tingling

6. Why do people with AIDS often suffer from anxiety and depression?

   a. AIDS is curable.

   b. Others may have negative attitudes about people with AIDS.

   c. Medications used to treat AIDS have pleasant side effects.

   d. People with AIDS often gain an enormous amount of weight.

Short Answer.

Mark the American Cancer Society's seven warning signs of cancer below with an "X."

7. _____ Change in bowel or bladder habits

8. _____ Difficulty breathing

9. _____ Dizziness

10. _____ Thickening or lump in breast or elsewhere

11. _____ Memory loss

12. _____ Obvious change in wart or mole

13. _____ Pain or swelling of the joints

14. _____ Nagging cough or persistent hoarseness

15. _____ Indigestion or difficulty swallowing

16. _____ Nausea or vomiting

17. _____ Sweet, fruity breath odor

18. _____ A sore that does not heal

19. _____ Unusual bleeding or discharge

20. _____ Headache

Briefly describe your role in caring for the resident with cancer regarding the items listed.

21. Communication

_____

_____

_____

_____

_____

_____

22. Nutrition

_____

_____

_____

_____

_____

_____

23. Pain control

_____

_____

_____

_____

_____

24. Comfort

_____

_____

_____

_____

_____

25. Skin care

_____

_____

_____

_____

26. Oral care

_____

_____

_____

_____

_____

_____

27. Self-image

_____

_____

_____

_____

_____

28. Psychosocial needs

_____

_____

_____

_____

_____

Unit 10. Describe mental illness, depression and related care

Scenarios.

Read each of the following scenarios, putting yourself in the resident's position, and then answer the questions for each scenario.

Annie, a nursing assistant, is taking care of a resident who is depressed. Annie is worried about Mrs. Rogers. She hurriedly dresses Mrs. Rogers even though Mrs. Rogers usually dresses herself. Annie says, "We don't want you to start crying today like you did yesterday."

1. What is Annie doing wrong?

_____

_____

_____

_____

_____

Bruce, a nursing assistant, is taking care of a mentally ill resident. The resident will sometimes yell at Bruce and accuse him of things. One day Bruce is helping the resident eat. The resident starts yelling: "I hate spaghetti. You always make me eat it, and it makes my stomach hurt. You want me to be sick! Leave me alone!"

2. Which of the following is the best response that Bruce can make?

a. "You have to eat this spaghetti because it's good for you."

b. "I'm sorry, I didn't realize you didn't like it. Would you like something else to eat instead?"

c. "You always say things like that. Of course you don't mean any of it. Just eat it, okay?"

d. "If you don't eat this, you won't get any dessert."

Name: _____

Word Search.

Complete each of the following sentences and find your answers in the word search.

3. Another term for lack of interest is

   _____ .

4. _____

   are an intense form of anxiety.

5. Manic depression is also called

   _____

   disorder.

6. Uneasiness or fear, often about a situation or condition.

   _____

7. When a person has a

   _____

   disorder, he or she is terrified for no known reason.

8. People cannot overcome depression through sheer _____ .

9. Obsessive behavior used to cope with anxiety is called

   _____

   disorder.

10. An NA should report to the nurse if a resident makes comments, even jokes, about hurting herself or others. Any threat of

   _____

   should be taken seriously.

y	f	m	b	c	o	w	k	x	d	k	z	p	q
o	l	h	s	j	b	w	j	r	j	p	h	k	i
j	e	l	g	v	s	b	r	a	l	o	p	i	b
x	n	a	w	x	e	p	t	w	b	g	p	d	a
b	p	a	v	o	s	p	x	i	v	a	g	d	a
d	c	f	w	k	s	e	a	p	f	a	m	y	k
t	u	e	q	n	i	s	l	o	o	s	h	e	r
k	v	j	z	d	v	w	p	h	s	t	e	x	w
j	y	l	d	k	e	y	n	y	a	e	x	q	c
p	a	n	i	c	c	r	t	p	z	z	m	f	e
d	e	k	u	y	o	m	a	e	h	i	w	s	d
r	d	k	f	i	m	b	p	c	i	o	c	o	c
g	i	z	i	b	p	w	z	d	k	x	x	z	s
x	c	r	v	z	u	a	w	y	w	y	n	q	j
n	i	h	x	a	l	w	r	y	u	y	h	a	d
m	u	h	j	t	s	d	i	a	h	x	g	g	z
t	s	d	s	s	i	q	i	l	y	g	f	g	i
o	e	e	j	e	v	f	p	w	l	u	d	o	w
j	y	s	u	s	e	b	l	u	h	t	i	n	j

nine

Rehabilitation and Restorative Services

Unit 1. Discuss rehabilitation and restorative care

Short Answer.

1. What is rehabilitation?

    _____

    _____

    _____

    _____

    _____

    _____

    _____

2. What are restorative services?

    _____

    _____

    _____

    _____

    _____

    _____

    _____

3. What are five important things that you should do during rehabilitation?

    _____

    _____

    _____

    _____

    _____

_____

_____

Unit 2. Describe the importance of promoting independence and list ways exercise improves health

Short Answer.

1. Why is it important for a resident to remain as independent as possible?

    _____

    _____

    _____

    _____

    _____

    _____

2. List five things that a lack of mobility may cause.

    _____

    _____

    _____

    _____

    _____

    _____

    _____

3. What are six factors that regular ambulation and exercise help improve?

    _____

    _____

Name: _____

_____
_____
_____
_____
_____

Unit 3. Describe assistive devices and equipment

Crossword.

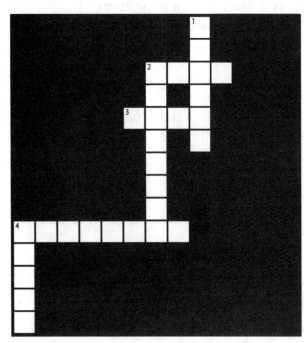

Clues:

Across

2. Adaptive equipment helps residents do these.

_____

3. Its purpose is to help with balance. Residents using one of these should be able to bear weight on both legs.

_____

4. These are used for residents who can bear no weight or limited weight on one leg.

_____

Down

1. It is used when the resident can bear some weight on the legs. It provides stability for residents who are unsteady or lack balance. _____

2. Type of devices that help people who are recovering from or adapting to a physical condition.

_____

4. Examples of personal care adaptive equipment are long-handled brushes and _____.

Unit 4. Describe positioning and how to assist with range of motion (ROM) exercises

Labeling.

Label each position below correctly.

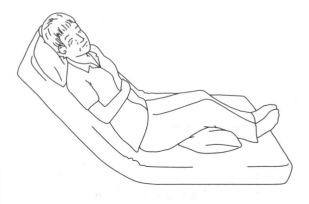

1. _____

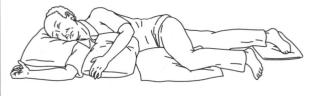

2. _____

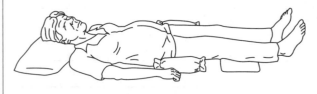

3. _____

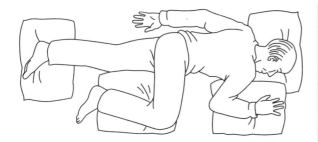

4. _____

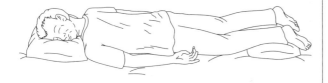

5. _____

Multiple Choice.

Circle the letter of the answer that best completes the statement or answers the question.

6. Helping residents into positions that are comfortable and healthy for them is called:
    a. Range of motion
    b. Positioning
    c. Massage
    d. Contractures

7. The device that is used to keep covers from resting on a resident's feet while in the supine position is called a:
    a. Splint
    b. Footboard
    c. Bed cradle
    d. Hand roll

8. A padded board placed against a resident's feet to keep them flexed is called a:
    a. Splint
    b. Footboard
    c. Bed cradle
    d. Hand roll

9. A device that is used to keep a resident's joints in the correct position is called a:
    a. Splint
    b. Footboard
    c. Bed cradle
    d. Hand roll

10. How often should nursing assistants help residents change positions to prevent pressure sores and stiffness?
    a. Every two hours
    b. Every five hours
    c. Every four hours
    d. Once per day

11. Which of the following means the permanent and painful stiffening of a joint and muscle and can result from lack of mobility?
    a. Range of motion
    b. Positioning
    c. Massage
    d. Contracture

Matching.

Write the letter of the correct definition beside each term listed below.

a. Turning downward

b. Moving a body part toward the body

c. Turning upward

d. Bending backward

e. Moving a body part away from the body

f. Straightening a body part

g. Bending a body part

h. Turning a joint

12. _____ Abduction

13. _____ Adduction

14. _____ Dorsiflexion

15. _____ Rotation

16. _____ Extension

17. _____ Flexion

18. _____ Pronation

19. _____ Supination

Labeling.

Correctly label each of the following movements used in range of motion exercises.

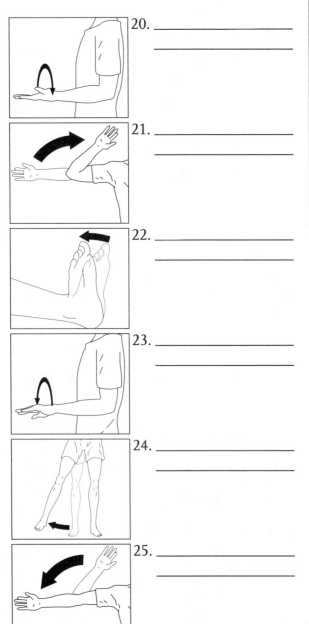

20. _____

21. _____

22. _____

23. _____

24. _____

25. _____

26. _____

27. _____

Unit 5. List guidelines for assisting with bowel and bladder retraining

Scenarios.

Read the following paragraphs and answer the questions.

Patty, a nursing assistant, sees that a resident has been incontinent. She says, "Oh no! You were doing so well until now."

1. What is wrong with Patty's reaction?

_____

_____

_____

_____

_____

_____

Tom, a nursing assistant, knows that a resident was incontinent last night. The resident asks Tom for a drink. Tom tells him, "You can't have any water now or you might have another accident."

2. What is wrong with Tom's reaction?

_____

_____

_____

_____

_____

_____

Name: _____

Jesse, a nursing assistant, enters a resident's room and begins giving her a long massage before bed. At the end of the massage, Jesse notices urine on the sheets.

3. What could Jesse have done that might have prevented this?

_____
_____
_____
_____
_____
_____
_____

Celia enters a resident's room and asks, "Is it time to change your diaper now?"

4. What is wrong with what Celia said?

_____
_____
_____
_____
_____
_____
_____

Unit 6. Describe care and use of prosthetic devices

True or False.

Mark each statement with either a "T" for true or an "F" for false.

1. _____ A prosthesis may replace an eye, arm, hand, foot, or leg.

2. _____ If you see that a prosthesis is cracked, try to repair it yourself.

3. _____ Prostheses are very expensive.

4. _____ A resident with a prosthesis will need special attention to help him adjust to changes.

5. _____ Phantom sensation is not real.

6. _____ You will be responsible for assisting a resident with a prosthesis with ADLs and ambulation.

7. _____ You should report any redness or open areas on a resident with a prosthesis.

8. _____ Phantom sensation should be treated as real pain and should not be ignored.

9. _____ It is not important to keep a prosthesis clean and dry.

10. _____ If the way a stump looks bothers you, you should tell the resident this.

11. _____ Artificial eyes should be cleaned with alcohol.

ten
Caring for Yourself

Unit 1. Describe how to find a job

Word Search.

Complete each of the following sentences and find your answers in the word search.

i	e	s	u	p	e	r	v	i	s	o	r	d	d
e	d	y	n	e	a	t	l	y	g	u	f	y	y
u	p	e	e	j	p	h	l	i	n	c	a	c	h
r	o	c	n	s	u	a	l	c	y	o	i	r	h
s	s	x	j	t	r	i	h	u	j	v	e	a	d
e	i	u	z	h	i	u	z	a	x	i	p	n	r
c	t	p	a	n	i	f	o	a	l	p	u	g	f
n	i	f	v	h	g	j	i	h	y	o	o	y	y
e	v	j	a	i	l	s	e	c	r	l	b	c	a
r	e	g	j	w	d	h	e	g	a	d	a	y	k
e	u	c	t	z	z	l	k	q	g	t	c	p	d
f	v	y	y	o	i	c	c	s	s	c	i	c	k
e	s	d	t	m	a	t	u	p	b	w	q	o	z
r	w	c	s	b	n	u	t	c	d	n	l	h	n

1. You should bring _____ with you to a job interview, such as a driver's license, social security card, passport, or birth certificate.

2. When arriving at a job interview, introduce yourself, _____, and shake hands.

3. _____ are people who can be called to recommend you as an employee.

4. Never _____ on a job application.

5. Be _____ when answering questions during a job interview. Emphasize what you enjoy about being a nursing assistant.

6. By law, your employer must perform a criminal _____ check. It is a law intended to protect residents.

7. Make sure you are dressed _____ and appropriately for a job interview.

8. During a job interview make _____ contact to show you are sincere.

9. Sit up or stand up straight, and look _____ to be at a job interview.

10. Questions you may want to ask during an interview include: Will my _____ be available when needed and what _____ would I work?

Short Answer.

11. Look at the illustration on the next page. This person is going to a job interview. What are some examples of how her appearance is unprofessional?

_____
_____
_____

Name: _____

_____
_____
_____
_____

Unit 2. Describe ways to be a great employee

Short Answer.

Samantha is a nursing assistant at Rolling Meadows Nursing Home. During one of her shifts, Samantha is called into her supervisor's office. Her supervisor says, "I've noticed that you've been late to work three times in a row. It's not fair to the other nursing assistants. And yesterday, you were unable to finish your assigned care tasks before your shift ended."

Samantha says, "I'm sorry I've been late. I've had a difficult time getting my son ready for school in the mornings. I'll make more of an effort to be on time. I know it's not fair to the others."

1. In this situation, what did Samantha do correctly?

_____
_____
_____
_____
_____
_____
_____

Jamie, a nursing assistant, walks into Mrs. Sandoval's room. Mrs. Sandoval's son and daughter are visiting her. When Jamie enters, Mrs. Sandoval's son walks over to her and yells, "It took you long enough to get here! My mother rang her call light 10 minutes ago. Are you too busy taking a break to get in here?"

Jamie says, "I got here as fast as I could. Why don't you just help her yourself if I'm so slow?"

2. In this situation, what did Jamie do incorrectly?

_____
_____
_____
_____
_____
_____
_____

Unit 3. Review guidelines for behaving professionally on the job

Mark a "P" next to all the examples of professional behavior below.

1. _____ Showing up for your shift 15 minutes late

2. _____ Wearing a uniform that has a stain on it

3. _____ Keeping your nails clean and trimmed

4. _____ Washing your hair and tying it back neatly

5. _____ Praising a resident for improvement in his abilities

6. _____ Not calling and not showing up for work

7. _____ Reporting a resident's new rash to the nurse

8. _____ Telling your supervisor, "I don't understand what that means. Can you please explain it?"

9. _____ Explaining a procedure to a resident before performing it

10. _____ Not telling a supervisor that a resident was in pain this morning

11. _____ Suggesting to your supervisor that you could take an agitated resident for a walk

Unit 4. Identify guidelines for maintaining certification and explain the state's registry

True or False.

Mark each statement with either a "T" for true or an "F" for false.

1. _____ OBRA requires that NAs complete at least 100 hours of training before being employed.

2. _____ Each state has the same requirements for maintaining NA certification.

3. _____ It is a good idea to know how long an absence from working as an NA is allowed without losing certification.

4. _____ Nursing assistants should respond quickly to their state's request to renew certification.

5. _____ NAs cannot add written statements to their files in the state registry.

6. _____ Each state keeps a registry for CNAs.

7. _____ Information about abuse and neglect becomes a part of an NA's permanent record in the state registry.

Unit 5. Describe continuing education for nursing assistants

True or False.

Mark each statement with either a "T" for true or an "F" for false.

1. _____ The federal government requires 20 hours of continuing education each year.

2. _____ Your responsibility for in-service education is to successfully attend and complete classes.

3. _____ Some states require more continuing education than the federal government.

4 _____ In-service continuing education courses help you keep your knowledge and skills fresh.

Short Answer.

5. List four of the responsibilities nursing assistants have for meeting continuing education requirements.

_____

_____

_____

_____

_____

_____

Name: _____

Unit 6. Define "stress" and "stressors" and explain ways to manage stress

Multiple Choice.

Circle the letter of the answer that best completes the statement or answers the question.

1. Which of the following statements is true of stress?

   a. Not managing stress does not cause problems.

   b. Stress is always caused by bad situations.

   c. Stress is an emotional and physical response.

   d. Everybody has the same tolerance level for stress.

2. When the heart beats fast in stressful situations, it can be a result of an increase of which hormone?

   a. Testosterone

   b. Estrogen

   c. Adrenaline

   d. Progesterone

3. Not managing stress can cause:

   a. Good relationships with residents

   b. Satisfaction with the workplace

   c. Abusive behavior toward residents

   d. Feeling well-rested

4. Which of the following behaviors helps manage stress?

   a. Poor nutrition

   b. Regular exercise

   c. Smoking cigarettes

   d. Sleeping only a few hours per night

5. Which of the following are appropriate people to turn to for help in managing stress?

   a. Residents

   b. Supervisors

   c. Residents' family members

   d. Residents' friends

Short Answer.

6. What are some of the things that make you experience stress? How do you react when you're stressed?

   _____

   _____

   _____

   _____

   _____

   _____

   _____

   _____

   _____

   _____

   _____

   _____

7. Write out your own personal stress management plan. Be sure to include things like diet, exercise, relaxation, entertainment, etc.

   _____

   _____

   _____

   _____

   _____

   _____

   _____

   _____

   _____

   _____

   _____

procedure checklists

Many certification skills evaluations list washing your hands as the final step. Although you will not necessarily be tested on documenting a procedure or reporting changes to the nurse, those final steps are included in these procedure checklists. These steps are important. In a facility, you will need to document every procedure you perform. You will also need to report any changes you notice while providing care. Always knock and wait for permission to enter before performing a procedure.

two

Foundations of Resident Care

Abdominal thrusts for the conscious person

✓ **Procedure Steps**

❑ 1. Stands behind person and brings arms under person's arms. Wraps arms around person's waist.

❑ 2. Makes a fist with one hand. Places flat, thumb side of the fist against person's abdomen, above the navel but below the breastbone.

❑ 3. Grasps the fist with other hand. Pulls both hands toward self and up, quickly and forcefully.

❑ 4. Repeats until object is pushed out or person loses consciousness.

Comments:

Shock

✓ **Procedure Steps**

❑ 1. Has the person lie down on her back unless bleeding from the mouth or vomiting.

❑ 2. Controls bleeding if bleeding occurs.

❑ 3. Checks pulse and respirations if possible.

❑ 4. Keeps person as calm and comfortable as possible.

❑ 5. Maintains normal body temperature.

❑ 6. Elevates the feet unless person has a head or abdominal injury, breathing difficulties, or a fractured bone or back.

❑ 7. Does not give person anything to eat or drink.

❑ 8. Calls for help immediately.

Comments:

Heart attack

✓ **Procedure Steps**

❑ 1. Calls or has someone call the nurse.

❑ 2. Places person in a comfortable position. Encourages him to rest. Reassures him that he will not be left alone.

❑ 3. Loosens clothing around the neck.

❑ 4. Does not give person liquids or food.

❑ 5. Monitors person's breathing and pulse. If breathing stops or person has no pulse, performs rescue breathing or CPR if trained and allowed to do so.

❑ 6. Stays with person until help arrives.

Comments:

Fainting

✓ Procedure Steps

❑ 1. Has person lie down or sit down before fainting occurs.

❑ 2. If person is in sitting position, has her bend forward and place her head between her knees. If person is lying flat on her back, elevates the legs.

❑ 3. Loosens any tight clothing.

❑ 4. Has person stay in position for at least five minutes after symptoms disappear.

❑ 5. Helps person get up slowly. Continues to observe her for symptoms of fainting. Stays with her until she feels better.

❑ 6. Reports the incident to the nurse.

Comments:

Seizures

✓ Procedure Steps

❑ 1. Lowers person to the floor.

❑ 2. Has someone call the nurse immediately. Does not leave person unless has to get medical help.

❑ 3. Moves furniture away to prevent injury. If a pillow is nearby, places it

under his head.

❑ 4. Does not try to restrain the person.

❑ 5. Does not force anything between the person's teeth. Does not place hands in person's mouth.

❑ 6. Does not give liquids or food.

❑ 7. When the seizure is over, checks breathing.

❑ 8. Reports the length of the seizure and observations to the nurse.

Comments:

Bleeding

✓ Procedure Steps

❑ 1. Puts on gloves.

❑ 2. Holds thick sterile pad, a clean pad, or a clean cloth, handkerchief, or towel against the wound.

❑ 3. Presses down hard directly on the bleeding wound until help arrives. Does not decrease pressure. Puts additional pads over the first pad if blood seeps through. Does not remove the first pad.

❑ 4. Raises the wound above the heart to slow down the bleeding if possible.

❑ 5. When bleeding is under control, secures the dressing to keep it in place. Checks person for symptoms of shock. Stays with person until help arrives.

❑ 6. Washes hands.

Comments:

Name: _____

Washing hands

✓ **Procedure Steps**

- ❑ 1. Identifies self by name. Identifies resident by name.
- ❑ 2. Turns on water at sink.
- ❑ 3. Angles arms down holding hands lower than elbows. Wets hands and wrists thoroughly.
- ❑ 4. Applies skin cleanser or soap to hands.
- ❑ 5. Lathers all surfaces of hands, wrists, and fingers, producing friction, for at least 15 seconds.
- ❑ 6. Cleans nails by rubbing them in palm of other hand.
- ❑ 7. Rinses all surfaces of wrists, hands, and fingers, keeping hands lower than the elbows and the fingertips down.
- ❑ 8. Uses clean, dry paper towel to dry all surfaces of hands, wrists, and fingers.
- ❑ 9. Uses clean, dry paper towel or knee to turn off faucet, without contaminating hands.
- ❑ 10. Disposes of used paper towel(s) in wastebasket immediately after shutting off faucet.

Comments:

Putting on gloves

✓ **Procedure Steps**

- ❑ 1. Washes hands.
- ❑ 2. If right-handed, slides one glove on left hand (reverse if left-handed).
- ❑ 3. With gloved hand, slides other hand into second glove.

- ❑ 4. Interlaces fingers to smooth out folds and create a comfortable fit.
- ❑ 5. Carefully looks for tears, holes, or spots. Replaces the glove if necessary.
- ❑ 6. If wearing a gown, pulls the cuff of the gloves over the sleeve of gown.

Comments:

Taking off gloves

✓ **Procedure Steps**

- ❑ 1. Touches only the outside of one glove and pulls the first glove off by pulling down from the cuff. Glove should be turned inside out as it comes off hand.
- ❑ 2. With ungloved hand, reaches two fingers inside the remaining glove. Does not touch any part of the outside.
- ❑ 3. Pulls down, turning this glove inside out and over the first glove. Should be holding one glove from its clean inner side; other glove should be inside it.
- ❑ 4. Disposes of gloves properly.
- ❑ 5. Washes hands.

Comments:

Putting on a gown

✓ **Procedure Steps**

- ❑ 1. Washes hands.
- ❑ 2. Opens gown without shaking it. Slips arms into the sleeves and pulls gown on.
- ❑ 3. Ties neck ties into a bow.

☐ 4. Reaching behind, pulls gown until it completely covers clothing. Ties the back ties.

Comments:

Putting on a mask and goggles

✓ Procedure Steps

☐ 1. Washes hands.

☐ 2. Picks up mask by top strings or elastic strap. Does not touch mask where it touches face.

☐ 3. Adjusts mask over nose and mouth. Ties top strings first, then bottom strings.

☐ 4. Puts on goggles.

Comments:

five
Personal Care Skills

Giving a complete bed bath

✓ Procedure Steps

☐ 1. Washes hands.

☐ 2. Identifies self by name. Identifies resident by name.

☐ 3. Explains procedure to resident. Speaks clearly, slowly, and directly. Maintains face-to-face contact whenever possible.

☐ 4. Provides for resident's privacy with curtain, screen, or door. Makes sure room is a comfortable temperature.

☐ 5. Adjusts bed to a safe working level.

☐ 6. Adjusts position of side rails to ensure resident safety at all times.

☐ 7. Places bath blanket or towel over resident. Asks resident to hold onto it while removing or folding back top bedding. Keeps resident covered with bath blanket (or top sheet).

☐ 8. Fills basin with warm water. Tests water temperature with thermometer or wrist. Water temperature should be 105° to 110° F. Has resident check water temperature. Adjusts if necessary.

☐ 9. Puts on gloves if resident has open wounds.

☐ 10. Asks and assists resident to participate in washing.

☐ 11. Uncovers only one part of the body at a time. Places a towel under the body part being washed.

☐ 12. Washes, rinses, and dries one part of the body at a time. Starts at the head. Works down, and completes front first.

Eyes and Face:

☐ Washes face with wet washcloth (no soap). Begins with the eye farther away from self. Washes inner aspect to outer aspect. Uses a different area of the washcloth for each eye. Washes the face from the middle outward. Uses firm but gentle strokes. Washes neck and ears and behind the ears. Rinses and pats dry.

Arms:

☐ Washes arm and underarm with a soapy washcloth. Uses long strokes from the shoulder to the elbow. Rinses and pats dry. Washes the elbow. Washes, rinses, and dries from the elbow down to the wrist.

Hands:

❏ Washes hand in a basin. Cleans under the nails with an orangewood stick or nail brush. Gives nail care. Repeats for the other hand. Applies lotion if ordered.

Chest:

❏ Places towel across resident's chest. Pulls blanket down to the waist. Lifts towel only enough to wash the chest. Rinses it and pats dry. For a female resident, washes, rinses, and dries breasts and under breasts.

Abdomen:

❏ Folds the blanket down so that it still covers pubic area. Washes the abdomen, rinses, and pats dry. Covers with towel. Pulls blanket up to resident's chin. Removes towel.

Legs and Feet:

❏ Exposes one leg. Places a towel under it. Washes the thigh. Uses long downward strokes. Rinses and pats dry. Does the same from the knee to the ankle.

❏ Places the foot into the basin. Washes the foot and between the toes. Rinses foot and pats dry. Gives nail care if it has been assigned. Repeats steps for the other leg and foot.

Back:

❏ Helps resident move to the center of the bed. Asks resident to turn onto his side so back is facing self. Washes back, neck, and buttocks with long, downward strokes. Rinses and pats dry.

❏ 13. If resident cannot provide perineal care, provides it. Puts on gloves if hasn't already been done.

❏ 14. Changes bath water. Washes, rinses, and dries perineal area. Works from front to back.

❏ *For a female resident:*

Washes the perineum with soap and water from front to back. Uses single strokes. Uses a clean area of washcloth or clean washcloth for each stroke. Wipes the center of the perineum, then each side. Spreads the labia majora, and wipes from front to back on each side. Rinses the area in the same way. Dries entire perineal area moving from front to back. Uses a blotting motion with towel. Asks resident to turn on her side. Washes, rinses, and dries buttocks and anal area. Cleanses anal area without contaminating the perineal area.

❏ *For a male resident:*

If resident is uncircumcised, pulls back the foreskin first. Gently pushes skin towards the base of penis.

Holds the penis by the shaft. Washes in a circular motion from the tip down to the base. Uses a clean area of washcloth or clean washcloth for each stroke. Rinses the penis. If resident is uncircumcised, gently returns foreskin to normal position. Then washes the scrotum and groin. Rinses and pats dry. Asks resident to turn on his side. Washes, rinses, and dries buttocks and anal area. Cleanses anal area without contaminating the perineal area.

❏ 15. Provides deodorant.

❏ 16. Removes and disposes of gloves properly.

❏ 17. Puts clean gown on resident. Assists with brushing or combing resident's hair. Makes resident comfortable and replaces bedding.

❏ 18. Returns bed to appropriate position. Removes privacy measures. Puts call light within resident's reach.

□ 19. Places soiled clothing and linens in proper containers.

□ 20. Empties, rinses, and wipes bath basin. Returns to proper storage.

□ 21. Washes hands.

□ 22. Reports any changes in resident.

□ 23. Documents procedure.

Comments:

Shampooing in bed

✓ **Procedure Steps**

□ 1. Washes hands.

□ 2. Identifies self by name. Identifies resident by name.

□ 3. Explains procedure to resident. Speaks clearly, slowly, and directly. Maintains face-to-face contact whenever possible.

□ 4. Provides for resident's privacy with curtain, screen, or door. Makes sure room is at a comfortable temperature.

□ 5. Adjusts bed to a safe working level. Locks bed wheels.

□ 6. Lowers head of bed. Removes pillow.

□ 7. Tests water temperature with thermometer or wrist. Water temperature should be 105° F. Has resident check water temperature. Adjusts if necessary.

□ 8. Raises the side rail farthest from self.

□ 9. Places the waterproof pad under resident's head and shoulders. Covers resident with bath blanket. Folds back the top sheet and blankets.

□ 10. Places collection container under resident's head (e.g., trough, basin).

Places one towel across resident's shoulders.

□ 11. Protects resident's eyes with dry washcloth.

□ 12. Wets hair and applies shampoo.

□ 13. Lathers and massages scalp with fingertips without scratching scalp.

□ 14. Rinses hair until water runs clear. Applies conditioner and rinses as directed.

□ 15. Covers resident's hair with clean towel. Dries face with washcloth.

□ 16. Removes trough and waterproof covering.

□ 17. Raises head of bed.

□ 18. Gently rubs the scalp and hair with the towel.

□ 19. Dries and combs resident's hair as resident prefers.

□ 20. Returns bed to appropriate level. Removes privacy measures.

□ 21. Puts call light within resident's reach.

□ 22. Empties, rinses, and wipes bath basin/pitcher. Returns to proper storage.

□ 23. Cleans comb/brush. Returns hair dryer and comb/brush to proper storage.

□ 24. Places soiled linen in proper container.

□ 25. Washes hands.

□ 26. Reports any changes in resident.

□ 27. Documents procedure.

Comments:

Giving a shower or a tub bath

✓ Procedure Steps

☐ 1. Washes hands.

☐ 2. Places equipment in shower or tub room. Cleans shower or tub area and shower chair.

☐ 3. Washes hands.

☐ 4. Identifies self by name. Identifies resident by name.

☐ 5. Explains procedure to resident. Speaks clearly, slowly, and directly. Maintains face-to-face contact whenever possible.

☐ 6. Provides for resident's privacy with curtain, screen, or door.

☐ 7. Helps resident to put on nonskid footwear. Transports resident to shower or tub room.

For a shower:

☐ 8. Places shower chair into position and locks wheels. Safely transfers resident into shower chair.

☐ 9. Turns on water. Tests water temperature with the thermometer. Water temperature should be no more than 105° F. Has the resident check water temperature.

For a tub bath:

☐ 8. Safely transfers resident onto chair.

☐ 9. Fills tub halfway with warm water. Tests water temperature with thermometer. Water temperature should be no more than 105° F. Has resident check water temperature.

Final steps for either procedure:

☐ 10. Puts on gloves.

☐ 11. Helps resident remove clothing and shoes.

☐ 12. Helps resident into shower or tub.

Puts shower chair into shower and locks wheels.

☐ 13. Stays with resident during procedure.

☐ 14. Lets resident wash as much as possible. Assists to wash the face.

☐ 15. Helps resident shampoo and rinse hair.

☐ 16. Helps to wash and rinse the entire body. Moves from head to toe.

☐ 17. Turns off water or drains tub. Covers resident until tub drains. Rolls resident out of shower or helps resident out of tub and onto a chair.

☐ 18. Gives resident towel(s) and helps to pat dry. Pats dry under the breasts, between skin folds, in the perineal area, and between toes.

☐ 19. Applies lotion and deodorant.

☐ 20. Places soiled clothing and linens in proper containers.

☐ 21. Removes gloves and disposes of them. Washes hands.

☐ 22. Helps resident dress and comb hair. Puts on nonskid footwear. Returns resident to room.

☐ 23. Makes resident comfortable. Places call light within resident's reach.

☐ 24. Reports any changes in resident.

☐ 25. Documents procedure.

Comments:

Providing fingernail care

✓ Procedure Steps

☐ 1. Washes hands.

☐ 2. Identifies self by name. Identifies resident by name.

❑ 3. Explains procedure to resident. Speaks clearly, slowly, and directly. Maintains face-to-face contact whenever possible.

❑ 4. Provides for resident's privacy with curtain, screen, or door.

❑ 5. Adjusts bed to a safe working level. Locks bed wheels.

❑ 6. Fills basin halfway with warm water. Tests water temperature with thermometer or wrist. Water temperature should be 105°F. Has resident check water temperature. Adjusts if necessary.

❑ 7. Soaks resident's nails in basin of water. Soaks all 10 fingertips for two to four minutes.

❑ 8. Removes hands. Washes hands with soapy washcloth. Rinses. Pats hands dry with towel, including between fingers.

❑ 9. Puts on gloves.

❑ 10. Removes dirt from under nails with orangewood stick.

❑ 11. Wipes orangewood stick on towel after each nail. Washes resident's hands again and dries them.

❑ 12. Grooms nails with file or emery board. Files in a curve.

❑ 13. Finishes with nails smooth and free of rough edges.

❑ 14. Applies lotion from fingertips to wrist.

❑ 15. Returns bed to appropriate level.

❑ 16. Puts call light within resident's reach.

❑ 17. Empties, rinses, and wipes basin. Returns to proper storage.

❑ 18. Disposes of soiled linen in proper container.

❑ 19. Removes and disposes of gloves.

❑ 20. Washes hands.

❑ 21. Reports any changes in resident.

❑ 22. Documents procedure.

Comments:

Providing foot care

✓ **Procedure Steps**

❑ 1. Washes hands.

❑ 2. Identifies self by name. Identifies resident by name.

❑ 3. Explains procedure to resident. Speaks clearly, slowly, and directly. Maintains face-to-face contact whenever possible.

❑ 4. Provides for resident's privacy with curtain, screen, or door.

❑ 5. Adjusts bed to a safe working level. Locks bed wheels.

❑ 6. Fills basin halfway with warm water. Tests water temperature with thermometer or wrist. Water temperature should be 105° F. Has resident check water temperature. Adjusts if necessary.

❑ 7. Places basin on the bath mat.

❑ 8. Removes socks. Completely submerges feet in water. Soaks feet for 5 to 10 minutes.

❑ 9. Removes one foot from water. Washes entire foot, including between the toes and around nail beds, with soapy washcloth.

❑ 10. Rinses entire foot, including between the toes.

❑ 11. Dries entire foot, including between the toes.

❑ 12. Repeats steps 9-11 for the other foot.

❑ 13. Puts lotion in hand. Warms it by rubbing hands together.

❑ 14. Massages lotion into entire foot, except between toes, removing any excess with a towel.

❑ 15. Assists resident to replace socks.

❑ 16. Returns bed to appropriate level.

❑ 17. Empties, rinses, and wipes basin. Returns to proper storage.

❑ 18. Disposes of soiled linen in proper container.

❑ 19. Puts call light within resident's reach.

❑ 20. Removes and disposes of gloves.

❑ 21. Washes hands.

❑ 22. Reports any changes in resident.

❑ 23. Documents procedure.

Comments:

Combing or brushing hair

✓ Procedure Steps

❑ 1. Washes hands.

❑ 2. Identifies self by name. Identifies resident by name.

❑ 3. Explains procedure to resident. Speaks clearly, slowly, and directly. Maintains face-to-face contact whenever possible.

❑ 4. Provides for resident's privacy with curtain, screen, or door.

❑ 5. Adjusts bed to safe working level. Locks bed wheels.

❑ 6. Raises head of bed so resident is sitting up. Places a towel under head or around shoulders.

❑ 7. Removes any hair pins, hair ties, and clips.

❑ 8. Removes tangles. Gently combs out from ends of hair to scalp.

❑ 9. Brushes two-inch sections of hair at a time. Brushes from roots to ends.

❑ 10. Styles hair in the way resident prefers. Avoids childish hairstyles. Offers mirror to resident.

❑ 11. Returns bed to appropriate level.

❑ 12. Puts call light within resident's reach.

❑ 13. Returns supplies to proper storage. Cleans hair from brush/comb.

❑ 14. Disposes of soiled linen in the proper container.

❑ 15. Washes hands.

❑ 16. Reports any changes in resident.

❑ 17. Documents procedure.

Comments:

Shaving a resident

✓ Procedure Steps

❑ 1. Washes hands.

❑ 2. Identifies self by name. Identifies resident by name.

❑ 3. Explains procedure to resident. Speaks clearly, slowly, and directly. Maintains face-to-face contact whenever possible.

❑ 4. Provides for resident's privacy with curtain, screen, or door.

❑ 5. Adjusts bed to safe level. Locks bed wheels.

❑ 6. Raises head of bed so resident is sitting up.

Shaving using a safety or disposable razor:

❑ 7. Fills basin halfway with warm water. Drapes towel under resident's chin.

❑ 8. Puts on gloves.

❑ 9. Moistens beard with warm washcloth. Puts shaving cream or soap over area.

❑ 10. Holds skin taut. Shaves beard in downward strokes on face and upward strokes on neck. Rinses razor often in warm water.

❑ 11. Offers mirror to resident.

❑ 12. Washes, rinses, and dries face after the shave. Applies after-shave lotion as requested.

❑ 13. Removes towel.

❑ 14. Removes gloves.

Shaving using an electric razor:

❑ 7. Drapes towel under resident's chin.

❑ 8. Puts on gloves.

❑ 9. Applies pre-shave lotion as resident wishes.

❑ 10. Holds skin taut. Shaves with smooth, even movements.

❑ 11. Offers mirror to resident.

❑ 12. Applies after-shave lotion as requested.

❑ 13. Removes towel.

❑ 14. Removes gloves.

Final steps:

❑ 15. Makes sure that resident and environment are free of loose hairs.

❑ 16. Returns bed to appropriate level.

❑ 17. Puts call light within resident's reach.

❑ 18. *For safety razor:* Rinses safety razor. *For disposable razor:* Disposes of a disposable razor in biohazard container.

For electric razor: Cleans head of electric razor. Removes whiskers from razor. Re-caps shaving head. Returns razor to case.

❑ 19. Returns supplies and equipment to proper storage.

❑ 20. Washes hands.

❑ 21. Reports any changes in resident.

❑ 22. Documents procedure.

Comments:

Providing oral care

✓ **Procedure Steps**

❑ 1. Washes hands.

❑ 2. Identifies self by name. Identifies resident by name.

❑ 3. Explains procedure to resident. Speaks clearly, slowly, and directly. Maintains face-to-face contact whenever possible.

❑ 4. Provides for resident's privacy with curtain, screen, or door.

❑ 5. Adjusts bed to a safe working level. Locks bed wheels. Makes sure resident is in an upright sitting position.

❑ 6. Puts on gloves.

❑ 7. Places towel across resident's chest.

❑ 8. Wets brush and puts on small amount of toothpaste.

❑ 9. Cleans entire mouth (including tongue and all surfaces of teeth). Uses gentle strokes. First brushes upper teeth, then lower teeth. Brushes back and forth.

❑ 10. Holds emesis basin to resident's chin.

11. Has resident rinse mouth with water and spit into emesis basin.

12. Wipes resident's mouth and removes towel.

13. Disposes of soiled linen in the proper container.

14. Cleans and returns supplies to proper storage.

15. Removes gloves. Disposes of gloves properly.

16. Returns bed to appropriate level.

17. Puts call light within resident's reach.

18. Washes hands.

19. Reports any problems with teeth, mouth, tongue, and lips.

20. Documents procedure.

Comments:

Flossing teeth

✓ **Procedure Steps**

1. Washes hands.

2. Identifies self by name. Identifies resident by name.

3. Explains procedure to resident. Speaks clearly, slowly, and directly. Maintains face-to-face contact whenever possible.

4. Provides for resident's privacy with curtain, screen, or door.

5. Adjusts the bed to a safe level. Locks bed wheels. Makes sure resident is in an upright sitting position.

6. Puts on gloves.

7. Wraps the ends of floss securely around each index finger.

8. Starting with the back teeth, places floss between teeth. Moves it down the surface of the tooth. Uses a gentle sawing motion. Continues to the gum line. At the gum line, curves the floss into a letter C. Slips it gently into the space between the gum and tooth. Then goes back up, scraping that side of the tooth. Repeats this on the side of the other tooth.

9. After every two teeth, unwinds floss from fingers. Moves it so clean area is used. Flosses all teeth.

10. Offers water to rinse the mouth.

11. Offers resident a face towel when done flossing all teeth.

12. Disposes of soiled linen in the proper container.

13. Cleans and returns supplies to proper storage.

14. Removes and disposes of gloves properly.

15. Returns bed to appropriate level.

16. Puts call light within resident's reach.

17. Washes hands.

18. Reports any problems with teeth, mouth, tongue, and lips.

19. Documents procedure.

Comments:

Cleaning and storing dentures

✓ **Procedure Steps**

1. Washes hands.

2. Puts on gloves.

3. Lines sink/basin with a towel(s) or fills sink with water.

❏ 4. Rinses dentures in cool running water before brushing them.

❏ 5. Applies toothpaste or cleanser to toothbrush.

❏ 6. Brushes dentures on all surfaces.

❏ 7. Rinses all surfaces of dentures under cool running water.

❏ 8. Rinses denture cup before placing clean dentures in it.

❏ 9. Places dentures in clean denture cup with solution or cool water. Makes sure cup is labeled with resident's name.

❏ 10. Cleans and returns the equipment to proper storage.

❏ 11. Disposes of towels in appropriate container or drains sink.

❏ 12. Removes and disposes of gloves properly.

❏ 13. Washes hands.

❏ 14. Reports any changes in appearance of dentures.

❏ 15. Documents procedure.

Comments:

Providing oral care for the unconscious resident

✓ **Procedure Steps**

❏ 1. Washes hands.

❏ 2. Identifies self by name. Identifies resident by name.

❏ 3. Explains procedure to resident. Speaks clearly, slowly, and directly. Maintains face-to-face contact whenever possible.

❏ 4. Provides for resident's privacy with curtain, screen, or door.

❏ 5. Adjusts bed to a safe level. Locks bed wheels.

❏ 6. Puts on gloves.

❏ 7. Turns resident's head to the side. Places a towel under his cheek and chin. Places an emesis basin next to the cheek and chin.

❏ 8. Holds mouth open with padded tongue blade.

❏ 9. Dips swab in cleaning solution. Wipes teeth, gums, tongue, and inside surfaces of mouth. Changes swab often. Repeats until the mouth is clean.

❏ 10. Rinses with clean swab dipped in water.

❏ 11. Removes the towel and basin. Pats lips or face dry if needed. Applies lip moisturizer.

❏ 12. Disposes of soiled linen in the proper container.

❏ 13. Cleans and returns supplies to proper storage.

❏ 14. Removes and disposes of gloves properly.

❏ 15. Returns bed to appropriate level.

❏ 16. Puts call light within resident's reach.

❏ 17. Washes hands.

❏ 18. Reports any changes in resident.

❏ 19. Documents procedure.

Comments:

Dressing a resident with an affected (weak) right arm

✓ **Procedure Steps**

- ❏ 1. Washes hands.
- ❏ 2. Identifies self by name. Identifies resident by name.
- ❏ 3. Explains procedure to resident. Speaks clearly, slowly, and directly. Maintains face-to-face contact whenever possible.
- ❏ 4. Provides for resident's privacy with curtain, screen, or door.
- ❏ 5. Asks resident which outfit she would like to wear. Dresses her in outfit of choice.
- ❏ 6. Removes resident's gown without completely exposing resident. Takes off stronger side first when undressing.
- ❏ 7. Assists resident to put the right (affected/weak) arm through the right sleeve of the shirt, sweater, or slip before placing garment on left (unaffected) arm.
- ❏ 8. Assists resident to put on skirt, pants, or dress.
- ❏ 9. Places bed at a safe level for resident, usually the lowest position.
- ❏ 10. Applies non-skid footwear. Ties laces.
- ❏ 11. Finishes with resident dressed appropriately. Makes sure clothing is right-side-out and zippers/buttons are fastened.
- ❏ 12. Places gown in soiled linen container.
- ❏ 13. Puts call light within resident's reach.
- ❏ 14. Washes hands.
- ❏ 15. Reports any changes in resident.
- ❏ 16. Documents procedure.

Comments:

Assisting resident with use of bedpan

✓ **Procedure Steps**

- ❏ 1. Washes hands.
- ❏ 2. Identifies self by name. Identifies resident by name.
- ❏ 3. Explains procedure to resident. Speaks clearly, slowly, and directly. Maintains face-to-face contact whenever possible.
- ❏ 4. Provides for resident's privacy with curtain, screen, or door.
- ❏ 5. Before placing bedpan, lowers head of bed. Locks bed wheels.
- ❏ 6. Applies gloves.
- ❏ 7. Covers resident with a bath blanket and pulls down covers underneath, not exposing more than necessary.
- ❏ 8. Places a protective pad under resident's buttocks and hips.
- ❏ 9. Asks resident to remove undergarments or helps him do so.
- ❏ 10. Places bedpan correctly under resident's buttocks (Standard bedpan: Positions bedpan so wider end of pan is aligned with resident's buttocks; Fracture pan: Positions bedpan with handle toward foot of bed).
- ❏ 11. Raises head of bed after placing bedpan under resident.
- ❏ 12. Puts toilet tissue within resident's reach.
- ❏ 13. Leaves call light within resident's reach while resident is using bedpan. Asks resident to signal when finished.

❑ 14. Returns and lowers head of bed.

❑ 15. Removes bedpan carefully. Covers bedpan.

❑ 16. Provides perineal care if assistance is needed.

❑ 17. Empties contents of bedpan into toilet. Notes color, odor, and consistency of contents.

❑ 18. Rinses bedpan, pouring rinse water into toilet, and uses disinfectant.

❑ 19. Removes and disposes of gloves properly.

❑ 20. Washes hands and puts on clean gloves.

❑ 21. Returns bedpan to proper storage.

❑ 22. Assists resident to wash hands. Disposes of soiled washcloth or wipes in proper container. Helps resident put on undergarment.

❑ 23. Removes and disposes of gloves properly.

❑ 24. Returns bed to appropriate level.

❑ 25. Puts call light within resident's reach.

❑ 26. Washes hands.

❑ 27. Reports any changes in resident.

❑ 28. Documents procedure.

Comments:

Assisting a male resident with a urinal

✓ **Procedure Steps**

❑ 1. Washes hands.

❑ 2. Identifies self by name. Identifies resident by name.

❑ 3. Explains procedure to resident. Speaks clearly, slowly, and directly.

Maintains face-to-face contact whenever possible.

❑ 4. Provides for resident's privacy with curtain, screen, or door.

❑ 5. Locks bed wheels. Puts on gloves.

❑ 6. Places a protective pad under resident's buttocks and hips.

❑ 7. Hands the urinal to resident. If resident is not able to help himself, places urinal between his legs and positions penis inside the urinal. Replaces bed covers.

❑ 8. Leaves call light within resident's reach. Asks resident to signal when finished.

❑ 9. Removes urinal; empties contents into toilet. Notes color, odor, and qualities of contents.

❑ 10. Rinses urinal, pouring rinse water into toilet. Uses disinfectant and returns to proper storage.

❑ 11. Removes and disposes of gloves.

❑ 12. Assists resident to wash hands. Disposes of soiled washcloth or wipes properly.

❑ 13. Puts call light within resident's reach.

❑ 14. Washes hands.

❑ 15. Reports any changes in resident.

❑ 16. Documents procedure.

Comments:

Helping a resident use a portable commode

✓ **Procedure Steps**

❑ 1. Washes hands.

❑ 2. Identifies self by name. Identifies resi-

Name: _____

dent by name.

☐ 3. Explains procedure to resident. Speaks clearly, slowly, and directly. Maintains face-to-face contact whenever possible.

☐ 4. Provides for resident's privacy with curtain, screen, or door.

☐ 5. Helps to portable commode. Makes sure resident is wearing non-skid shoes.

☐ 6. If needed, helps resident remove clothing and sit comfortably on toilet seat. Puts toilet tissue within resident's reach.

☐ 7. Leaves call light within resident's reach. Asks resident to signal when done.

☐ 8. Returns and puts on gloves.

☐ 9. Gives perineal care if help is needed.

☐ 10. Assists resident to wash hands. Disposes of soiled washcloth or wipes properly.

☐ 11. Assists resident back to bed.

☐ 12. Removes waste container and empties contents into toilet. Notes color, odor, and consistency of contents.

☐ 13. Rinses container, pouring rinse water into toilet. Uses disinfectant and returns to proper storage.

☐ 14. Removes and disposes of gloves properly.

☐ 15. Puts call light within resident's reach.

☐ 16. Washes hands.

☐ 17. Reports any changes in resident.

☐ 18. Documents procedure.

Comments:

Providing perineal care for an incontinent resident

✓ **Procedure Steps**

☐ 1. Washes hands.

☐ 2. Identifies self by name. Identifies resident by name.

☐ 3. Explains procedure to resident. Speaks clearly, slowly, and directly. Maintains face-to-face contact whenever possible.

☐ 4. Provides for resident's privacy with curtain, screen, or door.

☐ 5. Adjusts bed to a safe level. Locks bed wheels.

☐ 6. Lowers head of bed. Positions resident lying flat on his or her back. Raises side rail farthest from self.

☐ 7. Tests water temperature with thermometer or wrist. Water temperature should be 105° to 109° F. Has resident check water temperature. Adjusts if necessary.

☐ 8. Puts on gloves.

☐ 9. Covers resident with bath blanket. Moves top linens to foot of bed.

☐ 10. Removes soiled protective pad from underneath resident by turning resident on his side, away from self. Rolls soiled pad into itself with wet side in/dry side out.

☐ 11. Places clean protective pad under buttocks.

☐ 12. Returns resident to lying on his back.

☐ 13. Exposes perineal area only. Cleans perineal area.

☐ 14. Turns resident on his side away from self. Removes the wet protective pad after drying buttocks.

❏ 15. Places a dry protective pad underneath resident.

❏ 16. Repositions resident.

❏ 17. Replaces top covers. Removes bath blanket.

❏ 18. Places soiled linens, clothing, and protective pad in proper containers.

❏ 19. Empties, rinses, and wipes basin. Returns to proper storage.

❏ 20. Removes and disposes of gloves properly.

❏ 21. Returns bed to appropriate level.

❏ 22. Puts call light within resident's reach.

❏ 23. Washes hands.

❏ 24. Reports any changes in resident.

❏ 25. Documents procedure.

Comments:

Giving a back rub

✓ Procedure Steps

❏ 1. Washes hands.

❏ 2. Identifies self by name. Identifies resident by name.

❏ 3. Explains procedure to resident. Speaks clearly, slowly, and directly. Maintains face-to-face contact whenever possible.

❏ 4. Provides for resident's privacy with curtain, screen, or door.

❏ 5. Adjusts bed to a safe working level. Locks bed wheels.

❏ 6. Positions resident lying on his side or stomach. Covers with a cotton blanket. Exposes back to the top of the buttocks.

❏ 7. Warms lotion.

❏ 8. Places hands on each side of upper part of the buttocks. Makes long, smooth upward strokes with both hands along each side of the spine, up to the shoulders. Circles hands outward. Moves back along outer edges of the back. At buttocks, makes another circle and moves hands back up to the shoulders. Repeats this for three to five minutes without taking hands from resident's skin.

❏ 9. Kneads with the first two fingers and thumb of each hand. Places them at base of the spine. Moves upward together along each side of the spine. Applies gentle downward pressure with fingers and thumbs. Follows same direction as with the long smooth strokes, circling at shoulders and buttocks.

❏ 10. Gently massages bony areas (spine, shoulder blades, hip bones) with circular motions of fingertips.

❏ 11. Finishes with some long, smooth strokes.

❏ 12. Dries the back if extra lotion remains on it.

❏ 13. Removes blanket and towel.

❏ 14. Assists resident with getting dressed.

❏ 15. Stores supplies. Places soiled clothing and linens in proper containers.

❏ 16. Returns bed to appropriate level.

❏ 17. Puts call light within resident's reach.

❏ 18. Washes hands.

❏ 19. Reports any changes in resident.

❏ 20. Documents procedure.

Comments:

Name: _____

Assisting resident to move up in bed

✓ **Procedure Steps**

❑ 1. Washes hands.

❑ 2. Identifies self by name. Identifies resident by name.

❑ 3. Explains procedure to resident. Speaks clearly, slowly, and directly. Maintains face-to-face contact whenever possible.

❑ 4. Provides for resident's privacy with curtain, screen, or door.

❑ 5. Adjusts bed to a safe working level. Locks bed wheels.

❑ 6. Lowers head of bed. Moves pillow to head of the bed.

❑ 7. Lowers the side rail (if not already lowered) on side nearest self.

❑ 8. Stands alongside bed with feet apart, facing resident.

❑ 9. Places one arm under resident's shoulder blades and the other arm under resident's thighs.

❑ 10. Asks resident to bend knees, brace feet on mattress, and push feet on the count of three.

❑ 11. On signal, shifts body weight. Moves resident, while resident pushes with her feet.

❑ 12. Places pillow under resident's head.

❑ 13. Returns bed to appropriate level.

❑ 14. Puts call light within resident's reach.

❑ 15. Washes hands.

❑ 16. Reports any changes in resident.

❑ 17. Documents procedure.

Comments:

Moving a resident to the side of the bed

✓ **Procedure Steps**

❑ 1. Washes hands.

❑ 2. Identifies self by name. Identifies resident by name.

❑ 3. Explains procedure to resident. Speaks clearly, slowly, and directly. Maintains face-to-face contact whenever possible.

❑ 4. Provides for resident's privacy with curtain, screen, or door.

❑ 5. Adjusts bed to a safe working level. Locks bed wheels.

❑ 6. Lowers head of bed.

❑ 7. Gently slides hands under the head and shoulders and moves toward self. Gently slides hands under midsection and moves toward self. Gently slides hands under hips and legs and moves toward self.

❑ 8. Returns bed to appropriate level.

❑ 9. Puts call light within resident's reach.

❑ 10. Washes hands.

❑ 11. Reports any changes in resident.

❑ 12. Documents procedure.

Comments:

Turning a resident

✓ **Procedure Steps**

❑ 1. Washes hands.

❑ 2. Identifies self by name. Identifies resident by name.

❑ 3. Explains procedure to resident. Speaks clearly, slowly, and directly. Maintains face-to-face contact whenever possible.

Name: _____

❑ 4. Provides for resident's privacy with curtain, screen, or door.

❑ 5. Adjusts bed to a safe working level. Locks bed wheels.

❑ 6. Lowers head of bed.

❑ 7. Stands on side of bed opposite to where person will be turned. The far side rail should be raised.

❑ 8. Lowers side rail nearest self if it is up.

❑ 9. Moves resident to side of bed nearest self.

❑ 10. *Turning resident away from self:*

Crosses resident's arm over his chest. Crosses leg nearest self over far leg.

a. Stands with feet about 12 inches apart. Bends knees.

b. Places one hand on resident's shoulder and the other on resident's hip nearest self.

c. Gently pushes resident toward the other side of the bed. Shifts weight from back leg to front leg.

❑ *Turning resident toward self:*

Crosses resident's arm over his chest. Crosses leg furthest from self over near leg.

a. Raises both side rails.

b. Stands with feet about 12 inches apart. Bends knees.

c. Places one hand on resident's far shoulder and the other on resident's far hip.

d. Gently rolls resident toward self.

❑ 11. Positions resident properly. Proper body alignment requires:

❑ Head supported by pillow

❑ Shoulder adjusted so resident is not lying on arm

❑ Top arm supported by pillow

❑ Back supported by supportive device

❑ Top knee flexed

❑ Supportive device between legs with top knee flexed; knee and ankle supported

❑ 12. Returns bed to appropriate level.

❑ 13. Puts call light within resident's reach.

❑ 14. Washes hands.

❑ 15. Reports any changes in resident.

❑ 16. Documents procedure.

Comments:

Logrolling a resident with one assistant

✓ Procedure Steps

❑ 1. Washes hands.

❑ 2. Identifies self by name. Identifies resident by name.

❑ 3. Explains procedure to resident. Speaks clearly, slowly, and directly. Maintains face-to-face contact whenever possible.

❑ 4. Provides for resident's privacy with curtain, screen, or door.

❑ 5. Adjusts bed to a safe working level. Locks bed wheels.

❑ 6. Lowers the head of bed.

❑ 7. Lowers the side rail closest to self.

❑ 8. One person stands at resident's head and shoulders. The other stands near resident's midsection.

❑ 9. Places resident's arms across his or her chest. Places a pillow between the knees.

❏ 10. Stands with feet about 12 inches apart. Bends knees.

❏ 11. Grasps the draw sheet on the far side.

❏ 12. On the count of three, gently rolls resident toward self, turning resident as a unit.

❏ 13. Repositions resident comfortably.

❏ 14. Returns bed to appropriate level.

❏ 15. Puts call light within resident's reach.

❏ 16. Washes hands.

❏ 17. Reports any changes in resident.

❏ 18. Documents procedure.

Comments:

Assisting resident to sit up on side of bed: dangling

✓ Procedure Steps

❏ 1. Washes hands.

❏ 2. Identifies self by name. Identifies resident by name.

❏ 3. Explains procedure to resident. Speaks clearly, slowly, and directly. Maintains face-to-face contact whenever possible.

❏ 4. Provides for resident's privacy with curtain, screen, or door.

❏ 5. Adjusts bed height to lowest position. Locks bed wheels.

❏ 6. Raises the head of bed to sitting position.

❏ 7. Places one arm under resident's shoulder blades and the other arm under resident's thighs.

❏ 8. On the count of three, slowly turns resident into sitting position with legs dangling over side of bed.

❏ 9. Asks resident to hold onto edge of mattress with both hands. Assists resident to put on non-skid shoes.

❏ 10. Has resident dangle as long as ordered. Stays with resident at all times. Checks for dizziness. Helps resident lie down if dizzy and tells nurse.

❏ 11. Takes vital signs as ordered.

❏ 12. Removes slippers or shoes.

❏ 13. Gently assists resident back into bed. Places one arm around resident's shoulders. Places other arm under resident's knees. Slowly swings resident's legs onto bed.

❏ 14. Puts call light within resident's reach.

❏ 15. Washes hands.

❏ 16. Reports any changes in resident.

❏ 17. Documents procedure.

Comments:

Transferring a resident from bed to wheelchair

✓ Procedure Steps

❏ 1. Washes hands.

❏ 2. Identifies self by name. Identifies resident by name.

❏ 3. Explains procedure to resident. Speaks clearly, slowly, and directly. Maintains face-to-face contact whenever possible.

❏ 4. Provides for resident's privacy with curtain, screen, or door.

❏ 5. Removes footrests close to bed.

❏ 6. Places wheelchair near the head of

the bed with arm of the wheelchair almost touching the bed. Places wheelchair on resident's stronger, or unaffected, side.

❑ 7. Locks wheelchair wheels.

❑ 8. Raises head of the bed. Adjusts bed level to where the height is equal to or slightly higher than the chair. Locks bed wheels.

❑ 9. Assists resident to sitting position with feet flat on the floor.

❑ 10. Puts non-skid footwear on resident and securely fastens it.

❑ 11. *With transfer (gait) belt:*

   a. Stands in front of resident.

   b. Stands with feet about 12 inches apart. Bends knees.

   c. Places belt around resident's waist. Grasps belt on both sides.

Without transfer belt:

   a. Stands in front of resident.

   b. Stands with feet about 12 inches apart. Bends knees.

   c. Places arms around resident's torso under the arms.

❑ 12. Provides instructions to allow resident to help with transfer.

❑ 13. Counts to three to alert resident. On signal, slowly helps resident to stand.

❑ 14. Helps resident to pivot to front of wheelchair with back of resident's legs against wheelchair.

❑ 15. Lowers resident into wheelchair.

❑ 16. Repositions resident with hips touching back of wheelchair. Removes transfer belt, if used.

❑ 17. Attaches footrests. Places resident's feet on footrests.

❑ 18. Puts call light within resident's reach.

❑ 19. Washes hands.

❑ 20. Reports any changes in resident.

❑ 21. Documents procedure.

Comments:

Transferring a resident using a mechanical lift

✓ **Procedure Steps**

❑ 1. Washes hands.

❑ 2. Identifies self by name. Identifies resident by name.

❑ 3. Explains procedure to resident. Speaks clearly, slowly, and directly. Maintains face-to-face contact whenever possible.

❑ 4. Provides for resident's privacy with curtain, screen, or door.

❑ 5. Locks bed wheels.

❑ 6. Positions wheelchair next to bed. Locks brakes.

❑ 7. Helps resident to one side of the bed. Positions sling under resident, with the edge next to the resident's back. Makes the bottom of the sling even with resident's knees. Helps resident roll back to middle of bed. Spreads out edge of sling.

❑ 8. Rolls lift to bedside. Pushes base of lift under bed.

❑ 9. Places overhead bar directly over resident.

❑ 10. Attaches one set of straps to each side of the sling. Attaches one set of straps to overhead bar. Folds resident's arm across chest. Makes sure all straps are properly connected.

❑ 11. Raises resident two inches above the bed. Pauses for a moment to let resident gain balance.

❑ 12. Supports and guides resident's body. Moves the lift so that resident is positioned over the chair.

❑ 13. Slowly lowers resident into chair. Pushes down gently on resident's knees to help resident into sitting position.

❑ 14. Undoes straps from overhead bar. Leaves the sling in place.

❑ 15. Makes sure resident is seated comfortably.

❑ 16. Puts call light within resident's reach.

❑ 17. Washes hands.

❑ 18. Reports any changes in resident.

❑ 19. Documents procedure.

Comments:

six
Basic Nursing Skills

Admitting a resident

✓ Procedure Steps

❑ 1. Washes hands.

❑ 2. Identifies self by name. Identifies resident by name.

❑ 3. Explains procedure to resident. Speaks clearly, slowly, and directly. Maintains face-to-face contact whenever possible.

❑ 4. Provides for resident's privacy with curtain, screen, or door.

❑ 5. *If part of facility procedure, does the following:*

    ❑ Takes resident's height and weight.

    ❑ Takes resident's baseline vital signs.

    ❑ Obtains a urine specimen if required.

    ❑ Completes the paperwork, including an inventory of all the personal items.

    ❑ Helps resident to put personal items away.

    ❑ Provides fresh water.

❑ 6. Shows resident to the room and bathroom. Explains how to work equipment.

❑ 7. Introduces resident to roommate, other residents, and staff.

❑ 8. Puts call light within resident's reach.

❑ 9. Washes hands.

❑ 10. Documents procedure.

Comments:

Transferring a resident

✓ Procedure Steps

❑ 1. Washes hands.

❑ 2. Identifies self by name. Identifies resident by name.

❑ 3. Explains procedure to resident. Speaks clearly, slowly, and directly. Maintains face-to-face contact whenever possible.

❑ 4. Provides for resident's privacy with curtain, screen, or door.

❑ 5. Collects the items to be moved and takes them to the new location.

❑ 6. Helps resident into the wheelchair.

❑ 7. Introduces new residents and staff.

❑ 8. Assists resident to put personal items away.

❑ 9. Makes sure that resident is comfortable.

❑ 10. Puts call light within resident's reach.

❑ 11. Washes hands.

❑ 12. Reports any changes in resident.

❑ 13. Documents procedure.

Comments:

Discharging a resident

✓ Procedure Steps

❑ 1. Washes hands.

❑ 2. Identifies self by name. Identifies resident by name.

❑ 3. Explains procedure to resident. Speaks clearly, slowly, and directly. Maintains face-to-face contact whenever possible.

❑ 4. Provides for resident's privacy with curtain, screen, or door.

❑ 5. Compares the checklist to the items there. If all items are there, asks resident to sign.

❑ 6. Collects the items to be taken and takes them to pick-up area.

❑ 7. Helps resident dress and then helps resident into the wheelchair.

❑ 8. Helps resident to say good-byes to the staff and residents.

❑ 9. Transports resident to the pick-up area. Helps resident into vehicle.

❑ 10. Washes hands.

❑ 11. Documents procedure.

Comments:

Taking and recording oral temperature

✓ Procedure Steps

❑ 1. Washes hands.

❑ 2. Identifies self by name. Identifies resident by name.

❑ 3. Explains procedure to resident. Speaks clearly, slowly, and directly. Maintains face-to-face contact whenever possible.

❑ 4. Provides for resident's privacy with curtain, screen, or door.

❑ 5. Puts on gloves.

Using a mercury-free thermometer:

❑ 6. Holds thermometer by stem.

❑ 7. Shakes oral thermometer down to below the lowest number.

❑ 8. Puts on disposable sheath, if applicable. Inserts bulb end of oral thermometer into resident's mouth, under tongue and to one side.

❑ 9. Tells resident to hold oral thermometer in mouth with lips closed. Assists as necessary. Asks resident not to bite down or to talk.

❑ 10. Leaves thermometer in place for at least three minutes.

❑ 11. Removes the thermometer. Wipes with tissue from stem to bulb or removes sheath. Disposes of tissue or sheath.

❑ 12. Holds thermometer at eye level. Rotates until line appears. Rolls thermometer between thumb and forefinger. Reads temperature. Remembers temperature.

❏ 13. Rinses thermometer in warm water. Dries and returns it to plastic case or container.

Using a digital thermometer:

❏ 6. Puts on disposable sheath.

❏ 7. Turns on thermometer and waits until "ready" sign appears.

❏ 8. Inserts end of digital thermometer into resident's mouth, under tongue and to one side.

❏ 9. Leaves in place until thermometer blinks or beeps.

❏ 10. Removes the thermometer.

❏ 11. Reads temperature on display screen. Remembers temperature.

❏ 12. Using a tissue, removes and disposes of sheath.

❏ 13. Replaces thermometer in case.

Using an electronic thermometer:

❏ 6. Removes probe from base unit.

❏ 7. Puts on probe cover.

❏ 8. Inserts end of electronic thermometer into resident's mouth, under tongue and to one side.

❏ 9. Leaves in place until tone or light signals temperature has been read.

❏ 10. Reads temperature on display screen.

❏ 11. Removes the probe. Presses the eject button to discard the cover.

❏ 12. Remembers temperature.

❏ 13. Returns the probe to the holder.

Final steps:

❏ 14. Removes and disposes of gloves.

❏ 15. Immediately records name, temperature, date, time, and method used (oral).

❏ 16. Washes hands.

❏ 17. Puts call light within resident's reach.

❏ 18. Reports any changes in resident.

❏ 19. Documents procedure.

Comments:

Taking and recording rectal temperature

✓ **Procedure Steps**

❏ 1. Washes hands.

❏ 2. Identifies self by name. Identifies resident by name.

❏ 3. Explains procedure to resident. Speaks clearly, slowly, and directly. Maintains face-to-face contact whenever possible.

❏ 4. Provides for resident's privacy with curtain, screen, or door.

❏ 5. Adjusts bed to safe level. Locks bed wheels.

❏ 6. Helps resident to left-lying (Sims') position.

❏ 7. Folds back linens to expose only rectal area.

❏ 8. Puts on gloves.

❏ 9. *Mercury-free thermometer:* Holds thermometer by stem.

❏ *Digital thermometer:* Applies probe cover.

❏ 10. *Mercury-free thermometer:* Shakes thermometer down to below the lowest number.

❏ 11. Applies small amount of lubricant to bulb or probe cover.

❏ 12. Separates the buttocks. Gently inserts thermometer one inch into rectum.

❏ 13. Replaces sheet over buttocks. Holds on to the thermometer at all times.

❑ 14. *Mercury-free thermometer*: Holds thermometer in place for at least three minutes.

❑   *Digital thermometer*: Holds thermometer in place until thermometer blinks or beeps.

❑ 15. Removes the thermometer. Wipes with tissue from stem to bulb or removes sheath. Disposes of tissue or sheath.

❑ 16. Reads thermometer at eye level.

❑ 17. *Mercury-free thermometer*: Rinses thermometer and dries it. Returns it to plastic case or container.

❑   *Digital thermometer*: Throws away probe cover and returns thermometer to storage area.

❑ 18. Removes and disposes of gloves.

❑ 19. Immediately records name, temperature, date, time, and method used (rectal).

❑ 20. Washes hands.

❑ 21. Makes resident comfortable.

❑ 22. Places call light within reach.

❑ 23. Reports any changes in resident.

❑ 24. Documents procedure.

Comments:

Taking and recording tympanic temperature

✓ **Procedure Steps**

❑ 1. Washes hands.

❑ 2. Identifies self by name. Identifies resident by name.

❑ 3. Explains procedure to resident. Speaks clearly, slowly, and directly. Maintains face-to-face contact when-

ever possible.

❑ 4. Provides for resident's privacy with curtain, screen, or door.

❑ 5. Puts a disposable sheath over earpiece of the thermometer.

❑ 6. Straightens ear canal. Inserts covered probe into ear canal. Presses button.

❑ 7. Holds thermometer in place until thermometer blinks or beeps.

❑ 8. Reads temperature.

❑ 9. Disposes of sheath. Returns thermometer to storage or to charger.

❑ 10. Removes and disposes of gloves.

❑ 11. Immediately records name, temperature, date, time, and method used (tympanic).

❑ 12. Washes hands.

❑ 13. Puts call light within resident's reach.

❑ 14. Reports any changes in resident.

❑ 15. Documents procedure.

Comments:

Taking and recording axillary temperature

✓ **Procedure Steps**

❑ 1. Washes hands.

❑ 2. Identifies self by name. Identifies resident by name.

❑ 3. Explains procedure to resident. Speaks clearly, slowly, and directly. Maintains face-to-face contact whenever possible.

❑ 4. Provides for resident's privacy with curtain, screen, or door.

❑ 5. Adjusts bed to safe level. Locks bed wheels.

❑ 6. Removes resident arm from sleeve of gown. Wipes axillary area with tissues.

Using a mercury-free thermometer:

❑ 7. Holds thermometer at stem end and shakes down to below the lowest number.

❑ 8. Puts on disposable sheath, if applicable.

❑ 9. Places bulb end of thermometer in center of armpit and folds resident's arm over chest.

❑ 10. Holds in place for 10 minutes.

❑ 11. Removes the thermometer. Wipes with tissue from stem to bulb or removes sheath. Disposes of tissue or sheath.

❑ 12. Holds thermometer at eye level. Rotates until line appears. Reads temperature.

❑ 13. Cleans thermometer and/or returns it to container for used thermometers.

Using a digital thermometer:

❑ 7. Puts on disposable sheath. Turns on thermometer and waits until "ready" sign appears.

❑ 8. Positions end of thermometer in center of armpit and folds resident's arm over chest.

❑ 9. Holds in place until thermometer blinks or beeps.

❑ 10. Removes thermometer.

❑ 11. Reads temperature on display screen.

❑ 12. Removes and disposes of sheath with a tissue.

❑ 13. Replaces thermometer in case.

Using an electronic thermometer:

❑ 7. Removes probe from base unit.

❑ 8. Puts on probe cover.

❑ 9. Positions end of thermometer in center of armpit and folds resident's arm over chest.

❑ 10. Leaves in place until tone or light signals temperature has been read.

❑ 11. Reads the temperature on the display screen.

❑ 12. Removes the probe. Presses the eject button to discard the cover.

❑ 13. Returns the probe to the holder.

Final steps:

❑ 14. Puts resident's arm back into sleeve.

❑ 15. Removes and disposes of gloves.

❑ 16. Immediately records name, temperature, date, time, and method used (axillary).

❑ 17. Washes hands.

❑ 18. Puts call light within resident's reach.

❑ 19. Reports any changes in resident.

❑ 20. Documents procedure.

Comments:

Taking and recording radial pulse and counting and recording respirations

✓ Procedure Steps

❑ 1. Washes hands.

❑ 2. Identifies self by name. Identifies resident by name.

❑ 3. Explains procedure to resident. Speaks clearly, slowly, and directly. Maintains face-to-face contact whenever possible.

❑ 4. Provides for resident's privacy with curtain, screen, or door.

❏ 5. Places fingertips on thumb side of resident's wrist to locate pulse.

❏ 6. Counts beats for one full minute.

❏ 7. Keeping fingertips on resident's wrist, counts respirations for one full minute.

❏ 8. Records pulse rate, date, time and method used. Records respiratory rate and the pattern of breathing.

❏ 9. Puts call light within resident's reach.

❏ 10. Washes hands.

❏ 11. Reports any changes in resident to the nurse.

❏ 12. Documents procedure.

Comments:

Taking and recording blood pressure (one-step method)

✓ **Procedure Steps**

❏ 1. Washes hands.

❏ 2. Identifies self by name. Identifies resident by name.

❏ 3. Explains procedure to resident. Speaks clearly, slowly, and directly. Maintains face-to-face contact whenever possible.

❏ 4. Provides for resident's privacy with curtain, screen, or door.

❏ 5. Positions resident's arm with palm up. The arm should be level with the heart.

❏ 6. With the valve open, squeezes the cuff to make sure it is completely deflated.

❏ 7. Places blood pressure cuff snugly on resident's upper arm, with the center of the cuff placed over the brachial artery (1-1½ inches above the elbow

toward inside of elbow).

❏ 8. Wipes diaphragm and earpieces of stethoscope with alcohol wipes.

❏ 9. Locates brachial pulse with fingertips.

❏ 10. Places diaphragm of stethoscope over brachial artery.

❏ 11. Places earpieces of stethoscope in ears.

❏ 12. Closes the valve (clockwise) until it stops. Does not tighten it.

❏ 13. Inflates cuff to 30 mmHg above the point at which the pulse is last heard or felt.

❏ 14. Opens the valve slightly with thumb and index finger. Deflates cuff slowly.

❏ 15. Watches gauge. Listens for sound of pulse.

❏ 16. Remembers the reading at which the first clear pulse sound is heard. This is the systolic pressure.

❏ 17. Continues listening for a change of pulse sound. The point of change or when sound disappears is the diastolic pressure. Remembers reading.

❏ 18. Opens the valve to deflate cuff completely. Removes cuff.

❏ 19. Records both the systolic and diastolic pressures.

❏ 20. Wipes diaphragm and earpieces of stethoscope with alcohol. Stores equipment.

❏ 21. Puts call light within resident's reach.

❏ 22. Washes hands.

❏ 23. Reports any changes in resident.

❏ 24. Documents procedure.

Comments:

Taking and recording blood pressure (two-step method)

✓ **Procedure Steps**

❑ 1. Washes hands.

❑ 2. Identifies self by name. Identifies resident by name.

❑ 3. Explains procedure to resident. Speaks clearly, slowly, and directly. Maintains face-to-face contact whenever possible.

❑ 4. Provides for resident's privacy with curtain, screen, or door.

❑ 5. Positions resident's arm with palm up. The arm should be level with the heart.

❑ 6. With the valve open, squeezes the cuff to make sure it is completely deflated.

❑ 7. Places blood pressure cuff snugly on resident's upper arm, with the center of the cuff placed over the brachial artery (1-1½ inches above the elbow toward inside of elbow).

❑ 8. Locates the radial (wrist) pulse with fingertips.

❑ 9. Closes the valve (clockwise) until it stops. Inflates cuff, watching gauge.

❑ 10. Stops inflating cuff when pulse is no longer felt. Notes the reading. The number is an estimate of the systolic pressure.

❑ 11. Opens the valve to deflate cuff completely.

❑ 12. Writes down the systolic reading.

❑ 13. Wipes diaphragm and earpieces of stethoscope with alcohol wipes.

❑ 14. Locates brachial pulse with fingertips.

❑ 15. Places earpieces of stethoscope in ears.

❑ 16. Places diaphragm of stethoscope over brachial artery.

❑ 17. Closes the valve (clockwise) until it stops. Does not tighten it.

❑ 18. Inflates cuff to 30 mmHg above the estimated systolic pressure.

❑ 19. Opens the valve slightly with thumb and index finger. Deflates cuff slowly.

❑ 20. Watches gauge and listens for sound of pulse.

❑ 21. Remembers the reading at which the first clear pulse sound is heard. This is the systolic pressure.

❑ 22. Continues listening for a change or muffling of pulse sound. The point of a change or the point the sound disappears is the diastolic pressure. Remembers this reading.

❑ 23. Opens the valve to deflate cuff completely. Removes cuff.

❑ 24. Records both systolic and diastolic pressures.

❑ 25. Wipes diaphragm and earpieces of stethoscope with alcohol. Stores equipment.

❑ 26. Puts call light within resident's reach.

❑ 27. Washes hands.

❑ 28. Reports any changes in resident.

❑ 29. Documents procedure.

Comments:

Measuring and recording weight of an ambulatory resident

✓ **Procedure Steps**

❑ 1. Washes hands.

❑ 2. Identifies self by name. Identifies resident by name.

❑ 3. Explains procedure to resident. Speaks clearly, slowly, and directly. Maintains face-to-face contact whenever possible.

❑ 4. Provides for resident's privacy with curtain, screen, or door.

❑ 5. Starts with scale balanced at zero before weighing resident.

❑ 6. Helps resident to step onto the center of the scale.

❑ 7. Determines resident's weight.

❑ 8. Assists resident off scale before recording weight.

❑ 9. Records weight.

❑ 10. Puts call light within resident's reach.

❑ 11. Washes hands.

❑ 12. Reports any changes in resident.

❑ 13. Documents procedure.

Comments:

Measuring and recording height of an ambulatory resident

✓ Procedure Steps

❑ 1. Washes hands.

❑ 2. Identifies self by name. Identifies resident by name.

❑ 3. Explains procedure to resident. Speaks clearly, slowly, and directly. Maintains face-to-face contact whenever possible.

❑ 4. Provides for resident's privacy with curtain, screen, or door.

❑ 5. Assists resident to step onto scale, facing away from the scale.

❑ 6. Asks resident to stand straight. Helps as needed.

❑ 7. Pulls up measuring rod from back of scale. Gently lowers measuring rod until it rests flat on resident's head.

❑ 8. Determines resident's height.

❑ 9. Assists resident off scale before recording height.

❑ 10. Records height.

❑ 11. Puts call light within resident's reach.

❑ 12. Washes hands.

❑ 13. Reports any changes in resident.

❑ 14. Documents procedure.

Comments:

Measuring and recording urinary output

✓ Procedure Steps

❑ 1. Washes hands.

❑ 2. Puts on gloves before handling bedpan/urinal.

❑ 3. Pours the contents of the bedpan or urinal into measuring container. Does not spill or splash any of the urine.

❑ 4. Measures the amount of urine while keeping container level.

❑ 5. After measuring urine, empties measuring container into toilet. Does not splash.

❑ 6. Rinses measuring container and pours rinse water into toilet. Cleans container.

❑ 7. Rinses bedpan/urinal and pours rinse water into toilet. Uses disinfectant.

❑ 8. Returns bedpan/urinal and measuring container to proper storage.

❑ 9. Removes and disposes of gloves.

❏ 10. Washes hands before recording output.

❏ 11. Records contents of container in output column on sheet.

❏ 12. Reports any changes in resident.

Comments:

Providing catheter care

✓ **Procedure Steps**

❏ 1. Washes hands.

❏ 2. Identifies self by name. Identifies resident by name.

❏ 3. Explains procedure to resident. Speaks clearly, slowly, and directly. Maintains face-to-face contact whenever possible.

❏ 4. Provides for resident's privacy with curtain, screen, or door.

❏ 5. Adjusts bed to a safe working level. Locks bed wheels.

❏ 6. Lowers head of bed. Positions resident lying flat on her back. Raises the side rail farthest from self.

❏ 7. Removes or folds back top bedding, keeping resident covered with bath blanket.

❏ 8. Tests water temperature with thermometer or wrist. Water temperature should be 105° to 109° F. Has resident check water temperature. Adjusts if necessary.

❏ 9. Puts on gloves.

❏ 10. Asks resident to flex knees and raise her buttocks off the bed. Places clean protective pad under buttocks.

❏ 11. Exposes only the area necessary to clean the catheter.

❏ 12. Places towel or pad under catheter tubing before washing.

❏ 13. Applies soap to wet washcloth. Cleans area around meatus. Uses a clean area of washcloth for each stroke.

❏ 14. Holds catheter near meatus.

❏ 15. Cleans at least four inches of catheter nearest meatus. Moves in only one direction, away from meatus. Uses a clean area of the cloth for each stroke.

❏ 16. Rinses area around meatus, using a clean area of cloth for each stroke.

❏ 17. Rinses at least four inches of catheter nearest meatus. Moves in only one direction, away from meatus. Uses a clean area of the cloth for each stroke.

❏ 18. Replaces top covers. Removes bath blanket.

❏ 19. Disposes of linen in containers.

❏ 20. Empties, rinses, and wipes basin. Returns to proper storage.

❏ 21. Removes and disposes of gloves.

❏ 22. Returns bed to appropriate level.

❏ 23. Puts call light within resident's reach.

❏ 24. Washes hands.

❏ 25. Reports any changes in resident.

❏ 26. Documents procedure.

Comments:

Collecting a routine urine specimen

✓ **Procedure Steps**

❏ 1. Washes hands.

❏ 2. Identifies self by name. Identifies resident by name.

❏ 3. Explains procedure to resident. Speaks clearly, slowly, and directly.

Maintains face-to-face contact when-ever possible.

❏ 4. Provides for resident's privacy with curtain, screen, or door.

❏ 5. Puts on gloves.

❏ 6. Helps the resident to bathroom or commode or offers bedpan or urinal.

❏ 7. Has resident void. Asks resident not to put toilet paper in with sample. Provides a plastic bag for toilet paper.

❏ 8. Helps as necessary with perineal care. Helps resident wash his hands.

❏ 9. Takes bedpan to the bathroom.

❏ 10. Pours urine in specimen container, making sure container is at least half full.

❏ 11. Covers container with lid without touching the inside of container. Wipes off outside of container.

❏ 12. Places container in plastic bag.

❏ 13. Discards extra urine. Rinses and cleans equipment. Uses disinfectant. Stores.

❏ 14. Removes and disposes of gloves. Washes hands and helps resident to wash hands.

❏ 15. Completes the label for the container with resident's name, address, the date, and time.

❏ 16. Returns bed to proper position.

❏ 17. Puts call light within resident's reach.

❏ 18. Washes hands.

❏ 19. Reports any changes in resident.

❏ 20. Documents procedure. Notes amount and characteristics of urine.

Comments:

Collecting a clean catch (mid-stream) urine specimen

✓ **Procedure Steps**

❏ 1. Washes hands.

❏ 2. Identifies self by name. Identifies resident by name.

❏ 3. Explains procedure to resident. Speaks clearly, slowly, and directly. Maintains face-to-face contact when-ever possible.

❏ 4. Provides for resident's privacy with curtain, screen, or door.

❏ 5. Puts on gloves.

❏ 6. Opens the specimen kit. Does not touch the inside of the container or the inside of the lid.

❏ 7. Cleans perineal area properly if resident cannot do it on his or her own.

❏ 8. Asks resident to urinate into the bed-pan, urinal, or toilet, and to stop before urination is complete.

❏ 9. Places container under the urine stream and has resident start urinat-ing again. Fills the container at least half full. Has resident finish urinating in bedpan, urinal, or toilet.

❏ 10. Covers container with lid without touching the inside of container. Wipes off outside of container.

❏ 11. Places container in a plastic bag.

❏ 12. If using a bedpan or urinal, discards extra urine. Rinses and cleans equip-ment. Uses disinfectant. Stores.

❏ 13. Removes and disposes of gloves. Washes hands. Helps resident wash hands.

❏ 14. Completes the label for the container with resident's name, address, the date, and time.

□ 15. Puts call light within resident's reach.

□ 16. Washes hands.

□ 17. Reports any changes in resident.

□ 18. Documents procedure. Notes amount and characteristics of urine.

Comments:

Collecting a stool specimen

✓ **Procedure Steps**

□ 1. Washes hands.

□ 2. Identifies self by name. Identifies resident by name.

□ 3. Explains procedure to resident. Speaks clearly, slowly, and directly. Maintains face-to-face contact whenever possible.

□ 4. Provides for resident's privacy with curtain, screen, or door.

□ 5. Puts on gloves.

□ 6. When resident is ready to move bowels, asks him not to urinate at the same time and not to put toilet paper in with the sample. Provides a plastic bag for toilet paper.

□ 7. Fits specimen pan to toilet or commode, or provides resident with bedpan. Leaves the room. Asks resident to signal when finished with bowel movement. Makes sure call light is within resident's reach.

□ 8. After the bowel movement, helps as necessary with perineal care. Helps resident wash his or her hands. Makes resident comfortable. Removes gloves.

□ 9. Washes hands again.

□ 10. Puts on clean gloves.

□ 11. Using the two tongue blades, takes about two tablespoons of stool and puts it in the container. Covers it tightly.

□ 12. Wraps the tongue blades in toilet paper and throws them away. Empties the bedpan or container into the toilet. Cleans equipment. Uses disinfectant. Stores.

□ 13. Completes the label for the container with resident's name, address, the date, and time. Bags the specimen.

□ 14. Removes and disposes of gloves.

□ 15. Puts call light within resident's reach.

□ 16. Washes hands.

□ 17. Reports any changes in resident.

□ 18. Documents procedure. Notes amount and characteristics of stool.

Comments:

Making an occupied bed

✓ **Procedure Steps**

□ 1. Washes hands.

□ 2. Identifies self by name. Identifies resident by name.

□ 3. Explains procedure to resident. Speaks clearly, slowly, and directly. Maintains face-to-face contact whenever possible.

□ 4. Provides for resident's privacy with curtain, screen, or door.

□ 5. Places clean linen on clean surface within reach.

□ 6. Adjusts bed to a safe working level. Lowers head of bed. Locks bed wheels.

□ 7. Puts on gloves.

❑ 8. Loosens top linen from the end of the bed on working side. Unfolds bath blanket over top sheet. Removes top sheet.

❑ 9. Raises side rail on far side of bed. Goes to other side. Helps resident to turn onto side, moving away from self toward raised side rail.

❑ 10. Loosens bottom soiled linen on working side.

❑ 11. Rolls bottom soiled linen toward resident. Tucks it snugly against resident's back.

❑ 12. Places and tucks in clean bottom linen. Finishes with bottom sheet free of wrinkles. Makes hospital corners to keep bottom sheet wrinkle-free.

❑ 13. Smoothes bottom sheet out toward resident. Makes sure there are no extra wrinkles in mattress pad. Rolls extra material toward resident. Tucks it under resident's body.

❑ 14. Unfolds waterproof pad and centers it on bed. Tucks side nearest self under the mattress. Smoothes out toward resident. Tucks as it was done with sheet.

❑ 15. Places draw sheet on the bed. Tucks in on side closest to self, smoothes, and tucks as with other bedding.

❑ 16. Raises side rail nearest self. Goes to other side of bed and lowers side rail. Helps resident to turn onto clean bottom sheet.

❑ 17. Loosens soiled linen. Rolls linen from head to foot of bed. Avoids contact with skin or clothes. Places it in a hamper/bag, at foot of the bed, or in a chair.

❑ 18. Pulls and tucks in clean bottom linen, just like other side. Finishes with bottom sheet free of wrinkles.

❑ 19. Places resident on his back. Raises side rail.

❑ 20. Unfolds top sheet. Places it over resident. As resident holds top sheet, slips bath blanket out from underneath. Places it in hamper.

❑ 21. Places blanket over top sheet. Tucks the bottom edges of top sheet and blanket under bottom of mattress. Makes hospital corners on each side. Loosens top linens over resident's feet. Folds back top sheet over blanket at top of bed about six inches.

❑ 22. Removes pillow. Turns soiled pillowcase inside out when removing it. Changes pillowcase. Places pillow under resident's head with open end away from door.

❑ 23. Returns bed to appropriate level.

❑ 24. Disposes of soiled linen in the proper container.

❑ 25. Puts call light within resident's reach.

❑ 26. Removes gloves.

❑ 27. Washes hands.

❑ 28. Reports any changes in resident.

❑ 29. Documents procedure.

Comments:

Making an unoccupied bed

✓ **Procedure Steps**

❑ 1. Washes hands.

❑ 2. Places clean linen on clean surface within reach.

❑ 3. Adjusts bed to a safe working level. Puts bed in flattest position.

❑ 4. Puts on gloves.

❑ 5. Loosens soiled linen. Rolls soiled linen (soiled side inside) from head to foot of bed. Avoids contact with skin or clothes. Places it in a bag, at foot of the bed, or in chair.

❑ 6. Removes and disposes of gloves. Washes hands.

❑ 7. Remakes bed. Spreads mattress pad. Makes hospital corners to keep bottom sheet wrinkle-free. Puts on mattress protector and draw sheet. Smoothes and tucks under sides of bed.

❑ 8. Places top sheet and blanket over bed. Centers these, and tucks under end of bed. Makes hospital corners. Folds down top sheet over blanket about six inches. Folds both top sheet and blanket down.

❑ 9. Removes pillows and pillowcases. Puts on clean pillowcases. Replaces pillows.

❑ 10. Returns bed to appropriate level.

❑ 11. Disposes of soiled linen.

❑ 12. Washes hands.

❑ 13. Documents procedure.

Comments:

Changing a dry dressing using non-sterile technique

✓ **Procedure Steps**

❑ 1. Washes hands.

❑ 2. Identifies self by name. Identifies resident by name.

❑ 3. Explains procedure to resident. Speaks clearly, slowly, and directly. Maintains face-to-face contact whenever possible.

❑ 4. Provides for resident's privacy with curtain, screen, or door.

❑ 5. Cuts pieces of tape long enough to secure the dressing. Hangs tape on the edge of a table within reach. Opens four-inch gauze square package without touching gauze. Places the opened package on a flat surface.

❑ 6. Puts on gloves.

❑ 7. Removes soiled dressing by gently peeling tape toward the wound. Lifts dressing off the wound. Does not drag it over wound. Observes dressing for any odor. Notes color of the wound. Disposes of used dressing in proper container. Removes and disposes of gloves.

❑ 8. Puts on new gloves. Touching only outer edges of new four-inch gauze, removes it from package. Applies it to wound. Tapes gauze in place. Secures it firmly.

❑ 9. Removes and disposes of gloves properly.

❑ 10. Puts call light within resident's reach.

❑ 11. Washes hands.

❑ 12. Reports any changes in resident.

❑ 13. Documents procedure.

Comments:

seven
Nutrition and Hydration

Serving fresh water

✓ **Procedure Steps**

❑ 1. Washes hands.

2. Identifies self by name. Identifies resident by name.

3. Puts on gloves.

4. Scoops ice into water pitcher. Adds fresh water.

5. Uses and stores ice scoop properly.

6. Takes pitcher to resident.

7. Pours glass of water for resident. Leaves pitcher and glass at bedside.

8. Makes sure that pitcher and glass are light enough for resident to lift. Leaves a straw if resident desires.

9. Puts call light within resident's reach.

10. Removes gloves.

11. Washes hands.

Comments:

Feeding a resident who cannot feed self

✓ Procedure Steps

1. Washes hands.

2. Identifies self by name. Identifies resident by name.

3. Explains procedure to resident. Speaks clearly, slowly, and directly. Maintains face-to-face contact whenever possible.

4. Picks up diet card. Verifies that resident has received the right tray.

5. Assists resident to wash hands.

6. Adjusts bed height to put self at resident's eye level. Locks bed wheels.

7. Raises head of bed. Makes sure resident is in an upright sitting position.

8. Helps resident to put on clothing protector, if desired.

9. Sits facing resident. Sits at resident's eye level. Sits on stronger side.

10. Offers drink of beverage. Offers different types of food, allowing for resident's preferences.

11. Offers the food in bite-sized pieces.

12. Makes sure resident's mouth is empty before next bite or sip.

13. Offers beverage to resident throughout the meal.

14. Talks with resident during meal.

15. Wipes food from resident's mouth and hands as needed during the meal. Wipes again at the end of the meal.

16. Removes clothing protector if used. Disposes of in proper container.

17. Removes food tray. Checks for personal items.

18. Puts call light within resident's reach.

19. Washes hands.

20. Reports any changes in resident.

21. Documents procedure.

Comments:

eight

Common, Chronic, and Acute Conditions

Putting a knee-high elastic stocking on a resident

✓ Procedure Steps

1. Washes hands.

❏ 2. Identifies self by name. Identifies resident by name.

❏ 3. Explains procedure to resident. Speaks clearly, slowly, and directly. Maintains face-to-face contact whenever possible.

❏ 4. Provides for resident's privacy with curtain, screen, or door.

❏ 5. Turns stocking inside-out at least to heel area.

❏ 6. Gently places foot of stocking over toes, foot, and heel.

❏ 7. Gently pulls top of stocking over foot, heel, and leg.

❏ 8. Makes sure there are no twists or wrinkles in stocking after it is applied.

❏ 9. Puts call light within resident's reach.

❏ 10. Washes hands.

❏ 11. Reports any changes in resident.

❏ 12. Documents procedure.

Comments:

Caring for an ostomy

✓ **Procedure Steps**

❏ 1. Washes hands.

❏ 2. Identifies self by name. Identifies resident by name.

❏ 3. Explains procedure to resident. Speaks clearly, slowly, and directly. Maintains face-to-face contact whenever possible.

❏ 4. Provides for resident's privacy with curtain, screen, or door.

❏ 5. Adjusts bed to a safe working level.

❏ 6. Places protective sheet under resident. Covers resident with a bath blanket. Pulls down the top sheet and blankets. Only exposes ostomy site. Offers resident a towel to keep clothing dry.

❏ 7. Puts on gloves.

❏ 8. Removes ostomy bag carefully. Places it in plastic bag. Notes the color, odor, consistency, and amount of stool in the bag.

❏ 9. Wipes the area around the stoma with toilet paper. Discards paper in plastic bag.

❏ 10. Using a washcloth and warm soapy water, washes the area around the stoma, in one direction, away from the stoma. Pats dry with another towel. Applies cream as ordered.

❏ 11. Places the clean ostomy appliance on resident. Makes sure the bottom of the bag is clamped.

❏ 12. Removes disposable bed protector and discards. Places soiled linens in proper containers.

❏ 13. Removes bag. Discards bag in proper container.

❏ 14. Removes and disposes of gloves properly.

❏ 15. Puts call light within resident's reach.

❏ 16. Washes hands.

❏ 17. Reports any changes in resident.

❏ 18. Documents procedure.

Comments:

nine

Rehabilitation and Restorative Services

Assisting a resident to ambulate

✓ **Procedure Steps**

❑ 1. Washes hands.

❑ 2. Identifies self by name. Identifies resident by name.

❑ 3. Explains procedure to resident. Speaks clearly, slowly, and directly. Maintains face-to-face contact whenever possible.

❑ 4. Provides for resident's privacy with curtain, screen, or door.

❑ 5. Before ambulating, puts on and properly fastens non-skid footwear on resident.

❑ 6. Adjusts bed to lowest position. Locks bed wheels.

❑ 7. Stands in front of and faces resident.

❑ 8. Braces resident's lower extremities. Bends knees. Places one foot between resident's knees.

❑ 9. *With transfer (gait) belt*: Places belt around resident's waist. Grasps the belt, while assisting resident to stand.

❑ *Without transfer belt*: Places arms around resident's torso under resident's armpits, while assisting resident to stand.

❑ 10. *With transfer belt*: Walks slightly behind and to one side of resident for the full distance, while holding onto the transfer belt.

❑ *Without transfer belt*: Walks slightly behind and to one side of resident for the full distance, with arm supporting resident's back.

❑ 11. After ambulation, removes transfer belt if used. Assists resident to a comfortable position.

❑ 12. Returns bed to proper level.

❑ 13. Puts call light within resident's reach.

❑ 14. Washes hands.

❑ 15. Reports any changes in resident.

❑ 16. Documents procedure.

Comments:

Assisting with ambulation for a resident using a cane, walker, or crutches

✓ **Procedure Steps**

❑ 1. Washes hands.

❑ 2. Identifies self by name. Identifies resident by name.

❑ 3. Explains procedure to resident. Speaks clearly, slowly, and directly. Maintains face-to-face contact whenever possible.

❑ 4. Provides for resident's privacy with curtain, screen, or door.

❑ 5. Before ambulating, puts on and properly fastens non-skid footwear on resident.

❑ 6. Adjusts bed to lowest position so that feet are flat on the floor. Locks bed wheels.

❑ 7. Stands in front of and faces resident.

❑ 8. Braces resident's lower extremities. Bends knees. Places one foot between resident's knees.

❑ 9. Places transfer belt around resident's waist and grasps the belt, while assisting resident to stand.

☐ 10. Helps as needed with ambulation with cane, walker, or crutches.

☐ 11. Walks slightly behind and to one side of resident. Holds the transfer belt if one is used.

☐ 12. Watches for obstacles in resident's path. Encourages resident to look ahead, not down at his or her feet.

☐ 13. Encourages resident to rest if tired. Lets resident set the pace.

☐ 14. After ambulation, removes transfer belt. Assists resident to a position of comfort and safety.

☐ 15. Returns bed to appropriate level.

☐ 16. Puts call light within resident's reach.

☐ 17. Washes hands.

☐ 18. Reports any changes in resident.

☐ 19. Documents procedure.

Comments:

Assisting with passive range of motion exercises

✓ Procedure Steps

☐ 1. Washes hands.

☐ 2. Identifies self by name. Identifies resident by name.

☐ 3. Explains procedure to resident. Speaks clearly, slowly, and directly. Maintains face-to-face contact whenever possible.

☐ 4. Provides for resident's privacy with curtain, screen, or door.

☐ 5. Adjusts bed to a safe working level. Locks bed wheels.

☐ 6. Positions resident lying supine on the bed, with the body in good alignment.

☐ 7. Repeats each exercise at least three times.

☐ 8. Shoulder. Supports resident's arm at elbow and wrist. Performs the following exercises:
  - ☐ flexion/extension
  - ☐ abduction/adduction

☐ 9. Elbow. Performs the following exercises:
  - ☐ flexion
  - ☐ extension
  - ☐ pronation
  - ☐ supination

☐ 10. Wrist. Performs the following exercises:
  - ☐ flexion
  - ☐ extension
  - ☐ radial flexion
  - ☐ ulnar flexion

☐ 11. Thumb. Performs the following exercises:
  - ☐ abduction
  - ☐ adduction
  - ☐ opposition
  - ☐ flexion
  - ☐ extension

☐ 12. Fingers. Performs the following exercises:
  - ☐ flexion
  - ☐ extension
  - ☐ abduction
  - ☐ adduction

☐ 13. Hip. Performs the following exercises:
  - ☐ abduction
  - ☐ adduction
  - ☐ internal rotation
  - ☐ external rotation

❑ 14. Knees. Performs the following exercises:

    ❑   flexion

    ❑   extension

❑ 15. Ankles. Performs the following exercises:

    ❑   dorsiflexion

    ❑   plantar flexion

    ❑   supination

    ❑   pronation

❑ 16. Toes. Performs the following exercises:

    ❑   flexion and extension

    ❑   abduction

❑ 17. While supporting all limbs, moves all joints gently, slowly, and smoothly through the range of motion to the point of resistance. Stops if any pain occurs.

❑ 18. Returns bed to appropriate level.

❑ 19. Puts call light within resident's reach.

❑ 20. Washes hands.

❑ 21. Reports any changes in resident.

❑ 22. Documents procedure.

Comments: